MAKE SURE YOU
DO NOT HAVE
BREAST CANCER

MAKE SURE YOU DO NOT HAVE BREAST CANCER

PHILIP STRAX, M.D.

Introduction by Nancy Reagan

Foreword by Rose Kushner

St. Martin's Press / New York

MAKE SURE YOU DO NOT HAVE BREAST CANCER. Copyright © 1989
by Philip Strax, M.D. All rights reserved. Printed in the United
States of America. No part of this book may be used or
reproduced in any manner whatsoever without written permission
except in the case of brief quotations embodied in critical articles
or reviews. For information, address St. Martin's Press, 175 Fifth
Avenue, New York, N.Y. 10010.

Design by Karin Batten

Library of Congress Cataloging-in-Publication Data

Strax, Philip.
    Make sure you do not have breast cancer / Philip Strax : with a
foreword by Rose Kushner.
        p. cm.
    ISBN 0-312-03392-3
    1. Breast—Cancer—Popular works. I. Title.
RC280.B8S76   1989
616.99'449—dc20   89–35119

First Edition

10 9 8 7 6 5 4 3 2 1

This book is dedicated to the three and a half million volunteers of the American Cancer Society who give of themselves to further the prevention, early detection, and adequate treatment of cancer, as well as to the rehabilitation of the cancer patient.

This book is also dedicated to the many who are doing the same in other organizations on a national level, such as the U.O.T.S.(United Order True Sisters), as well as to organizations operating on the local scene, such as the Stella and Charles Guttman Breast Diagnostic Institute in New York City, and the Gertrude and Philip Strax Breast Cancer Detection Institute in Lauderhill, Florida.

These inspired and dedicated volunteers have learned that the greatest benefit in doing for others accrues to themselves. They echo the call: We must all strive together to conquer cancer in our lifetime!

OUR GOAL

The feminine breast has intrigued mere man
As a valuable, lovable, marvelous sight.
As a matter of fact, from the time man began
He's found it the source of much varied delight.

To all it brings life when life struggles to start
And then it excites ever more with the years.
To some it's a symbol of beauty and art,
To others it's sorrow and sadness and tears.

Perhaps if we X-ray and scrutinize well,
This wonderful structure well fashioned to nurse
May carry the clue in its succulent shell
To help us unravel the cancerous curse!

P.S.

CONTENTS

Contents

ACKNOWLEDGMENTS

I acknowledge with gratitude and appreciation the inspiration and help given me by Arthur I. Holleb, M.D., former first vice-president in charge of medical affairs, American Cancer Society; Nathaniel I. Berlin, M.D., former scientific director of biology and diagnosis, National Cancer Institute, whose foresight is helping to prevent needless deaths of women from breast cancer; and Joan Kahn, the original editor of *Early Detection*.

This book would never have been written without the encouragement and aid of my late wife Gertrude and my friends Virginia and Richard Adloff. Any success that this writing may have in furthering the motto of the Guttman Institute—"Early Detection Saves Lives— It May Save Yours!"—is due as much to their efforts as to mine.

The proceeds from the sale of this book will be divided between the Stella and Charles Guttman Breast Diagnostic Institute in New York City and the Gertrude and Philip Strax Breast Cancer Detection Institute in Lauderhill, Florida, and the American Cancer Society.

INTRODUCTION

Breast cancer had always been a faraway thought. But in Octobr 1987 I was faced with the realization that breast cancer had stricken me.

Being a doctor's daughter, regular checkups have always been an important part of my life. The mammogram that I had in October of 1987 detected a lump that had not been found through regular examination. By early detection and proper treatment, I live to share my thoughts with you today.

I was amazed—almost shocked—at the number of people I knew who had breast cancer and hadn't mentioned it until my story was on the front pages of the daily papers. It was very reassuring for me to talk to these people about their surgery and postoperative experiences, and they gave me a wonderful sense of hope and security for my own recovery. In addition, the thousands upon thousands of letters I received from strangers who became friends was like getting a special dose of medicine. They wrote to tell me that I was not alone. They had recovered and were leading happy, active lives. They shared wonderful stories and anecdotes—some filled with tears and many filled with laughter. But all filled with hope and promise.

Too many women today still live in darkness when it comes to breast cancer. It is too easy not to face the reality that it can happen to you. Dr. Philip Strax of the Guttman Institute of New York City and the Strax Institute of Florida has helped women all across the country to cope with the obstacles of breast cancer. His philosophy parallels mine in that he stresses the importance of regular medical checkups for early detection and prevention. He believes that education is crucial to a woman for both her mental and physical well-being.

Awareness of the precautions and procedures surrounding breast cancer is the first step in fighting the disease, and perhaps in taking this step, the number of lives lost to breast cancer could be reduced. This book concentrates on awareness, early detection, and education. I encourage all women to read this book. For the few minutes it takes one to read through these pages, many years may be added to one's life through absorbing the valuable information contained in this book.

It has been almost two years since my breast surgery and I have never felt better. My activities have not changed in any way. I feel wonderful and my husband tells me every day that he loves me more than the day we were married. A woman can't ask for more than that.

NANCY REAGAN

FOREWORD

In 1974, when Dr. Philip Strax published the first edition of *Early Detection: Breast Cancer Is Curable*, X-raying the breasts by mammography to see if cancer is present was still "experimental." Few doctors, and even fewer women, had ever heard of the miraculous machinery that can peer into a woman's breast and find a malignant tumor when it's only a microscopic cluster of cells. Yet in 1989, as I introduce this second book, *Make Sure You Do Not Have Breast Cancer*, I wouldn't be surprised if the only doctors and women who still don't know about mammography are recent immigrants from the planet Mars. Such procedures have become so accepted that, on July 1, 1988, President Ronald Reagan signed a law ordering Medicare to pay for its use for "screening"— the first disease-prevention legislation ever passed by the U.S. Congress.

In only fifteen years—a blink of the eye in the long history of medicine—Dr. Philip Strax, almost single-handedly, has made *mammography* a household world.

But this is jumping ahead of the Phil Strax story.

I accidentally found the tiny lump next to the nipple of my left breast in June, 1974, before Betty Ford and Happy Rockefeller so courageously publicized their mastectomies later that year. After their surgeries made front-page headlines around the world, the disease was literally pulled "out of the closet."

The words "breast cancer" were finally mentionable in polite society, breast self-examination (BSE) and mammography were demonstrated on prime-time television, and, by a happy coincidence, the first edition of *Early Detection* was published.

Unfortunately, however, none of these events helped me in June that year when I found my lump. I, like most women, knew nothing about breast cancer except that if the disease were diagnosed, the offending breast would automatically be amputated while I was asleep on the operating-room table. After my doctor examined my breast, he sent me to be X-rayed by a "newfangled gadget," mammography, that our local hospital had recently bought.

I soon learned that mammography was not newfangled at all: It had been available since the 1930s. Why wasn't it used routinely? Until 1974, most women waited until their breast cancers were so advanced that X rays weren't needed to make the diagnosis! Not until the wives of the President and Vice-President of the United States were treated four decades later did the impetus for early detection of breast cancer by BSE and mammography really begin.

But I am again jumping ahead of the Phil Strax story.

In 1962, when he was working with the Health Insurance Plan (HIP) in New York, Dr. Strax decided to prove scientifically that mammography could, indeed, save women's lives by detecting cancers of the breast before they were palpable—before they could be felt. More than 60,000 members of HIP—a prepaid health-maintenance organization—were randomly assigned as two carefully matched groups: one a "control" group to be examined routinely if any breast symptoms developed, and the other a "screened" group to be checked initially and then on an annual basis for three years by the standard physical examination plus mammography. All the women were presumably "asymptomatic," without symptoms of breast cancer. By 1969, it was becoming clear that those women who had unsuspected cancers detected in the screened group were living longer than those with cancers in the control group.

The early findings were impressive enough to persuade the American Cancer Society (ACS) and the National Cancer Institute (NCI) to fund a national screening program throughout the United States. Known as the Breast Cancer Detection Demonstration Project (BCDDP), the program began in 1973 and screened more than 280,000 women by the time it ended in 1979. Again, as with the now-legendary "HIP study," BCDDP data are proving that those women who were screened by mammography—and diagnosed and treated earlier—are living longer.

Dr. Strax's goal has never been to use breast X rays to diagnose cancer *after* a lump or other abnormality has been found; his goal has always been to use mammography to find cancers of the breast *before* they are palpable. For more than thirty years, he has devoted all of his time to convincing women, doctors, employers, and governments that detecting and treating breast cancers when the tumors are visible only on mammography will save millions of lives.

On June 15, 1988, Philip Strax—together with his HIP collaborator, Sam Shapiro—was awarded the prestigious General Motors Cancer Research Prize for his efforts on behalf of women. Thanks to Dr. Strax's foresight, tenacity, perseverance, and downright stubbornness, a screening examination by mammography is now recommended to be a routine for all women older than forty years of age.

We women owe him a debt that even General Motors can't repay for us. In this brief account of his long and difficult struggle, I want to thank him—although the word seems puny and inadequate—on behalf of all women for all he has done to reduce the terrible toll of breast cancer on our lives.

ROSE KUSHNER
Executive Director
Breast Cancer Advisory Center
Kensington, Maryland

PREFACE:
WHY THIS BOOK?

A similar book was first published in 1974 under the title *Early Detection: Breast Cancer Is Curable*. It served as a clarion call to women, primarily those over the age of thirty, to alert them to the hidden dragon in their midst —breast cancer—which was waiting to pounce on them without warning. The book was an attempt to warn all women that breast cancer could be present without any signs or symptoms at all. However, it emphasized the optimistic note that weapons were available that could detect the disease at a very early stage when the disease could be eradicated and a potential cure obtained.

The book was very well received, and was considered by many to be revolutionary for its time. It was translated into Dutch and Hebrew, among other languages. A special edition was sent out by the Book-of-the-Month Club to its subscribers *pro bono publico*. It stimulated many women to take advantage of the modern methods of detection of breast cancer then available. It undoubtedly led to the saving of many thousands of women's lives.

The book was based primarily on preliminary data from the Health Insurance Plan study, initiated by the author with the invaluable cooperation of Sam Shapiro, an epidemiologist, that indicated a substantial saving of lives from breast cancer through early detection. However, two further aspects of the problem needed to be looked into. The present book, *Make Sure You Do Not Have Breast Cancer*, addresses these problems.

In the first place, the Health Insurance Plan data in the early 1970s were rather preliminary. A long follow-up of the women in the study was needed to convince the medical profession that data had been produced that determined conclusively that lives could indeed be saved by early detection. We now have eighteen years of follow-up data that show without question that lives can be saved from breast cancer in the vast majority of cases *if the disease is detected early,* before signs or symptoms are present. Other studies, in Sweden and Holland, have corroborated these findings. It was felt that this valuable information could be used to further motivate women to take advantage of our weapons—especially since improved, more efficient methods of detection of breast cancer were now available.

Also, it has become more apparent that, despite great medical progress, only a small minority of women, even in 1989, are aware of the need and willing to accept the new procedures. Even more, a large proportion of the medical profession has yet to be convinced, and motivated to, in turn, urge women to follow through.

When we consider that a method for prevention of the disease still eludes us; when we consider that methods for cure of the disease at all stages—particularly the usual case when the disease has spread beyond the confines of the breast—are still not available; when we consider that our only effective method for control—and potential cure—is detection of the disease at a really early stage and that we now have the means to reach this goal, then the need for another clarion call to alert women to the danger they face and the protection that is available to them becomes more and more obvious.

This new revised and medically updated edition of

the original book is a vigorous attempt to once again make women aware of the dragon in their midst, of the need to destroy it before it destroys them, and of the availability of our new weapons to accomplish the deed.

A NOTE TO
THE READER

I have been involved, since 1960, in promoting my concept of early detection of breast cancer as a practical and important way of saving lives of women from this disease. My effort started with the initiation of a study involving the Health Insurance Plan of Greater New York. It was well conceived and well coordinated, particularly by my colleague, Sam Shapiro, an epidemiologist. It involved an examination of presumably well women to detect breast cancer by adding to the usual clinical examination the X-ray procedure called mammography (which had been available for many years, but hardly used) as a means for detecting the disease before it could be suspected or felt by even the most expert hands.

The concept, with the important help of Wanda Venet, R.N., and Louis Venet, M.D., led to the now internationally acclaimed HIP study. By now, we have achieved results of an eighteen-year follow-up of the study, which have proved conclusively that the screening or examining of presumably well women can lead to a substantial (25 percent) reduction in the death rate from breast cancer. In other words, a mechanism has been developed that can save at least one-quarter more women from breast cancer than was previously thought possible. The concept and the function of the study were recognized in 1988 with the awarding to Shapiro and myself of the highly prestigious General Motors Cancer Research Prize (the Charles F. Kettering Prize).

My original book, *Early Detection: Breast Cancer Is Curable*, was written when the early results of this study were promising. They led to the formation of the Stella and Charles Guttman Breast Diagnostic Institute in New York City and subsequently to a satellite center, the Gertrude and Philip Strax Breast Cancer Detection Institute in Lauderhill, Florida. The goal of the institutes was to pass along the potential benefits of screening to the general public, to develop improved techniques, and to stimulate motivation of women to accept the only proven method we have to reduce mortality from the disease. A large Breast Cancer Detection Demonstration Project (BCDDP), conducted by the American Cancer Society and the National Cancer Institute, was started in 1973 to evaluate motivation in women in some twenty-eight other centers across the United States. All the centers showed similar beneficial results and all showed potential for motivation of women to accept mass screening.

The original book was part of the attempt to stimulate women to accept the concept and come in for examinations, and to inform physicians of the potential of screening so that they in turn could motivate women. We have made considerable progress in this regard. The eighteen-year follow-up, with the persistent reduction in mortality, has, of course, been very helpful in convincing both the women and their physicians. Many screening centers have been developed in many areas, and our ongoing attempt to stimulate awareness of the problem has had increasing success. But there is still much to do. In spite of all our efforts to date, probably fewer than 25 percent of women over the age of thirty-five have ever had a mammogram to detect unsuspected disease.

This book is an essential step in our campaign. It has two important goals:

1. To reassure women that nine out of ten women will *not* develop breast cancer, and that the vast majority of women undergoing the complete examination will get the benefit of reassurance that the breasts are normal.
2. To reassure women that, in the event screening detects a small problem in the early stages, there is every likelihood that not only will a life be saved, but less surgery will be needed and a breast may be saved as well.

Many people, including physicians, think that the increase in numbers of women with breast cancer in the 1980s means that we are having a breast-cancer epidemic. Although it is true that in the past fifteen years we have had an increase in frequency of the disease from 1 in 15 to 1 in 10, it is also true that nine out of ten women today will not get breast cancer. There surely is no epidemic of the disease.

There surely is, however, *an epidemic of fear* of developing breast cancer. Very many women over twenty seem to have some preoccupation with the possibility of having or getting the disease. Most women have some breast discomfort at some time. Most women are conscious of tenderness or lumpiness. Most women are exposed to proliferation of information about breast cancer. The stories of prominent women who have developed the disease, like Betty Ford, Ann Jillian, and Nancy Reagan, and some of the painful accounts described vividly by writers like Betty Rollin, who have themselves been victims, have served to frighten women in general and particularly those exposed to the disease in family or friends.

What we need during this perceived period of crisis is reassurance that the vast majority of women *do not have and will not get the disease.* Women in general need a thorough examination for reassurance that all is well. Women need the peace of mind that follows such a complete, thorough examination to reassure them that no cancer is present. This examination must be done in a most professional manner by physicians and technicians aware of the concern and fear that the average woman has. The examination must be done in a gentle, sympathetic, and compassionate manner. Each woman needs to be reassured that the simple, quick, gentle, and painless examination of a presumably well woman leads, in the vast majority of cases, to a reassuring, completely negative report. Every woman needs to know that only a handful of cancers are found in a thousand presumably well women. Women must also be made aware that they need such reassurance on a regular, periodic basis (which is usually once a year) to make sure that they stay well and that no new problem has developed. They need to be reassured that under such a regime, if anything does turn up, it may require further study with a simple needle or a simple incision to be sure that no cancer is present. They must be reassured that if a cancer does turn up, it will be detected in an early, most likely curable stage that will require a simple operative procedure without removal of the breast. Early detection can save a life *and* a breast—and *that* is our goal!

MAKE SURE YOU DO NOT HAVE BREAST CANCER

1

DON'T BE AFRAID OF BREAST CANCER

The chances are ten to one that you will never get breast cancer. Furthermore, if you do, and have followed the simple precepts in this book, the chances are three out of four that your cancer will be detected in a curable stage, even at the present state of our knowledge—and our knowledge of this disease is increasing all the time.

Is breast cancer common? Emphatically, no! What is common is the *fear* of breast cancer. It is this fear that keeps many women from helping themselves by having breast examinations or even examining their own breasts. Our fight must be against this fear as well as against breast cancer itself.

It is true that most of us have been exposed to the miseries of breast cancer in close relatives, friends, or acquaintances. It is true that most women develop breast symptoms or even lumps at some time or other. It is true that many women who do develop the disease delay going to a physician until it is too late. But it is also true that only infrequently do such breast symptoms or lumps mean cancer. And it is also true that you can protect yourself by learning what breast cancer is all about and by following a few simple rules.

You must say to yourself: "I will most likely never get breast cancer, but if I do, I want to be in a position to overcome it!" That is the message of this book.

You will learn why women are so afraid of breast cancer, what it is, who will get it, how we find it, and what you can do to protect yourself against it. Read carefully, follow through—and don't be afraid!

We live in a breast-oriented society. To the average woman, her breast is the badge of femininity, an important part of her allure to charm her male. To the man, the breast is a source of excitement and erotic stimulation. It has become a bridge between male and female and is used as a reward to be flaunted before the eyes of the male in the female's attempt to attract him. This emphasis on the breast as a sex symbol begins in adolescence and apparently persists throughout life.

The problem of breast cancer is a double one: the cancer itself and perhaps equally important, the fact that the breast is involved. Of course, the most dreadful of all diseases to a woman is breast cancer. The specter of this disease hovers like a black cloud over all her thoughts and hopes. For many years, breast cancer wasn't even mentioned in news media, as though it were a stigma. The word "breast," referring to that important part of the female anatomy that we have all been intimately acquainted with from the time of birth, seemed to be taboo. A conspiracy of silence seemed to surround this remarkable feminine structure as though its existence were a myth. In recent years, thanks to efforts on the part of forward-seeing women and physicians, especially those of the American Cancer Society, the women of our society have become increasingly aware of the importance of the breast in the health of a woman, and the need for constant vigilance against the possibility of trouble.

Consider the following typical incidents, which occurred in one day in the life of a physician interested in breast conditions:

"I'm a schoolteacher in a supervisory position," said an attractive forty-five-year-old woman. "I first noticed this lump in my left breast two and a half years ago. At first, I thought it would just go away. It didn't hurt or bother me in any way. Then as I watched it get bigger and produce changes in the skin, I thought it was probably serious. I felt strongly about breast surgery and the fear of losing my breast. I simply couldn't bring myself to see a physician. I even wear a bra at night to hide the condition from my husband."

Mrs. Hammer was shifting uneasily in her chair. "Tell him, Gayle. You tell him about the lump." Gayle was obviously distraught and couldn't manage to communicate. Finally she blurted out: "I've got this small lump in my breast. I know it's nothing. Do you think I may have to lose my breast?"

My secretary was buzzing frantically. "Mrs. Weil out here is so nervous I think her teeth are chattering. She whispers something about a lump in her breast and she's really frightened. Please see her soon."

"Sit right here and talk to me," I said to the forty-two-year-old woman. "Why are you so hesitant?"

"Doctor," she began, "I know I'm cystic. Three doctors have told me that I have what sounds like cystic mastitis. It sounds terrible to me. I feel I have a serious disease that is progressing and will lead to my losing a breast. What can I do to prevent this happening?"

Mrs. K. lowered her eyes, clasped her hands, and began shyly. "My husband likes to manipulate my breasts as part of our lovemaking. Sometimes he's rather vigorous and once my breast was black and blue. I've heard that an injury can lead to cancer. Is that true? I've been worrying about our relationship."

The common thread in all these episodes is the tremendous preoccupation with the female breast that has been developing in the past forty years. Billboards, movie marquees, newspaper ads, and magazine photos all stress the female breast as the sex symbol of our age. All this is a far cry from the situation seventy years ago, when young developing breasts were strapped and tightened with vise-like brassieres, in an attempt to hide this womanly attribute from the predatory male's gaze.

This elevation of the female breast as an important sex attribute has brought with it a greater apprehension and anxiety about breast conditions. All women from early childhood have heard gruesome stories about serious breast diseases that led to all types of surgery. And the totally erroneous idea has been spreading among many women that the loss of a breast is equivalent to loss of sexual attraction or prowess or both. In short, a pathological national anxiety bordering on hysteria has come into existence in regard to the breast. Is it any wonder, then, that concern about breast diseases has reached alarming proportions and that a small, nontender lump or a pain or a discharge can produce a state of abject terror?

Unfortunately, it is true that breast cancer is a dangerous, troublesome, worrisome disease today. For instance:

- Every six minutes, breast cancer is diagnosed in the United States and every twelve minutes a woman dies of the disease.
- One of every four cancers in women is in the breast, so that this organ is the most common of all cancer sites.
- Breast cancer is the most common cause of death in women aged thirty-nine to forty-four.
- The chances of developing the disease increase throughout a woman's life, and the rate of development is much greater at seventy than it is at forty.
- We have really made no progress in this disease since 1930, as far as saving lives is concerned. Even today, up to one-third of patients with breast cancer are really inoperable when first seen. Of the remainder, less than one-half are alive and well ten years later. In

other words, despite all our surgical, radiotherapeutic, and chemotherapeutic techniques, we are probably curing only about 25 percent of women who present themselves to their physicians with this disease—and all because most breast cancer seen by the medical community is late cancer.

Add to this information the fact that even in the most expert hands three of every four breast operations show a benign condition. If it were known definitely that no cancer was present, the operation, called a *biopsy*, would not need to be done. It is, of course, proper that such a "look-see" procedure be carried out to make sure that cancer is not present, but the fact remains that the operation generates apprehension and concern. In some institutions where the clinician's expertise may be less or his own anxiety greater, more than nine out of ten operations may fall into this benign category. The sum of it all is that, although only one woman out of ten develops breast cancer, it is also true that many develop a condition warranting an operation, with all the concern it brings. Most women are then conditioned and concerned about their breasts for the rest of their lives, awaiting and often expecting the worst.

But the sun is beginning to show through the dark clouds, and a brighter tomorrow is beginning to dawn. The new hope is based on the following information:

It has long been known that if at the time of a breast cancer operation the local glands in the armpit (the axillary lymph nodes) are free of disease, meaning that the cancer is localized or confined to the breast, better than four out of five such women will be alive and well five years later. If, however, the glands are involved, not much more than one out of two will remain well.

Since cancer is a progressive disease that grows and usually spreads to the neighboring glands or through the bloodstream, it seems obvious that in order to improve the present situation, we must find breast cancers when they are still confined to the breast, before they have spread. We must engage in what is called *early detection*.

This concept is not new—it has been with us for many years. It has been the cornerstone of a major educational program of the American Cancer Society. It has been the reason for the ongoing campaign of that society for breast self-examination—to watch for the warning signals of cancer, such as a lump. But, unfortunately, the campaign has had slow success. Educational drives and advice to physicians to teach breast self-examination have not caused the death rate from breast cancer to decline. Over the years, some medical prophets of doom have felt that the fate of a woman who develops a breast cancer is sealed at the time of the appearance of the growth—that the outcome of the disease depends solely on the virulence of the cancer and the resistance of the woman's body. They have indicated that earlier detection was merely a way of finding the condition earlier, thus producing an apparent improvement equal to the period of early detection, but that the end result was the same.

What was needed in this controversy was proof—statistical proof—that earlier detection of breast cancer could indeed result in saving more lives, and not merely lead to increased survival from the time of diagnosis. The bright star on the horizon today is that such evidence is now at hand. How this evidence was obtained is an exciting story which we will go into subsequently. Suffice it to say here that in eighteen years of follow-up of two large matched groups of women it has been proved statistically that a reduction of almost one-third in the mortality rate was achieved in the group that received special examinations as compared with the group that did not. A method is today available that can save the lives of perhaps 30,000 of the 40,000 women who now die every year of breast cancer in the United States.

Another hope is also becoming apparent. Many surgeons, in various areas of the United States, like Dr. Bernard Fisher in Pittsburgh, and many others abroad feel that in those cancers found in the early stages— when small and localized in the breast—lesser surgery can achieve results as good as the more extensive kind needed for more advanced disease.

One of the dilemmas of breast cancer involves detection. We know that the earlier we find the disease the better are our results. We also pride ourselves as physicians that our training and knowledge permit us to diagnose medical conditions more easily and even before our patients discover them. Yet it is common knowledge that well over 90 percent of breast cancer is detected by the woman and not by her physician. Why do we rely on the woman to become aware of a condition that is curable in its early stages?

Physicians are trained to treat disease. They spend many hard years learning the intricacies of the normal structure and function of the human body and the abnormal changes we call disease. They learn to recognize the abnormalities and apply the appropriate treatment. Over the years there has been an increasing awareness of the value of the old Chinese concept that the worth of a physician can be measured more by his ability to keep you well than by his ability to make you whole—

that much pain and suffering could be avoided if body derangements were detected in the earliest stages, when less drastic measures would be needed for correction. This concept has reached its acme in "screening" for disease. This means setting up standards, like sieves, checking people to see how they measure up, and sifting out those with abnormalities. Of course, it also means getting people to accept the concept and to present themselves before a derangement makes itself known —before symptoms or signs of disease are present. It also means a heightened awareness on the part of the physician of the earliest signs of disease and a dedication to be willing to screen many people to find disease in only a few. It means a new orientation on the part of one who has been trained to treat disease when it exists. It also means that a physician must say to himself: "Examining many well people can be boring and hardly satisfying. However, the thought that every once in a while I'll find unsuspected disease at a stage when it is curable and thus perhaps save a life makes the whole business worthwhile." Fortunately, breast cancer falls into such a category.

The new era that is dawning in breast cancer thus means saving of lives and perhaps less radical surgical procedures for very early cancers. Someday the medical profession will be able to offer our girl babies the promise of immunity from breast cancer. Someday we may have the magic remedy that will cure the disease wherever it may have spread in the body and at whatever stage it may be. Until that time, let us use the remedies at hand that can save most of the women who become afflicted with this disease.

2

ALERTNESS COULD SAVE YOUR LIFE

Probably the most important breakthrough in breast cancer in the last thirty-five years has been the realization that earlier detection can result in lowered mortality from the disease—that finding the cancer earlier can save lives. This hopeful premise was developed as a result of three known but apparently unrelated facts.

1. Over 90 percent of breast cancer is detected by the woman herself. She finds her lump or "tumor," becomes uneasy, rushes to her physician after more or less delay while she hopes the abnormal mass will disappear, and tells him that last week or last night she found this little lump and "Of course, it does not bother me

and so it's nothing. Right?" Her physician is faced with a very apprehensive woman whom he would like to reassure. He is often under considerable pressure to follow a wait-and-see attitude with what may be a questionable lump. Eventually, if the mass is a definite and persistent one, it will be brought to the hands of a surgeon who will remove it and make a definite diagnosis.

It is, however, the woman herself who starts the train of events as the result of a lump or pain or nipple discharge. These days, when women realize more and more the value of a regular, complete physical examination with a Pap smear (named after its developer, Dr. Papanicolaou) to evaluate the neck of the womb, it is common for the gynecologist or other clinician to examine the breast routinely, and significant trouble is sometimes discovered in this way. Occasionally an abnormality is detected in the course of a screening examination offered with the specific purpose of finding a breast cancer earlier.

2. It has been known for many years that, regardless of how extensive a surgical procedure has been performed or whether X-ray or cobalt therapy has been used in conjunction with surgery, if there has been no involvement of glands in the armpit (known as axillary lymph nodes) at time of surgery, over 85 percent of the women will be alive and well five years after surgery. If, however, such glands have been involved with cancer, only about 50 percent will remain well. The obvious conclusion must be that the overwhelming factor determining the outcome is the extent of the disease at the time of operation. If the cancer is localized to the breast, the outcome is far more favorable. If the process has extended beyond the breast, the chances of complete recovery are far fewer. The lesson to be learned is: "Find

the cancer when it is still only in the breast, the earlier the better."

This concept, however, needed proof. Perhaps, it could be argued, those cancers that turned out to have no glandular involvement were actually milder cases. Perhaps, it was said, the overall death rate would be the same. Indeed, there had been mass screening examinations at cancer-detection centers using clinical examination only with very little effect on the mortality rate. Something else was needed.

3.   That something was the procedure known as mammography. This examination, which is merely a simple X-ray study of the breast without injection of any material and with only minimal handling of the breast, has a history extending back practically to the discovery of X rays at the very end of the last century. The first authenticated use of the procedure was in 1913. Over the years it had been advocated as a useful examination in France, Germany, Italy, the United States, and particularly Uruguay, where Dr. Raoul Leborgne emphasized its value in making breast-cancer diagnosis more accurate. He also clearly described X-ray findings of cancers before they could be felt. Although there was a flurry of activity in the 1930s and 1940s in the United States, the technique was discarded by most physicians for its uncertain results. Its praises continued to be sung, however, by Dr. Jacob Gershon-Cohen in Philadelphia, by Prof. Charles Gros in Strasbourg, and Dr. Leborgne in Montevideo, in addition to others in different parts of the world. As a matter of fact, mammography continued to be used increasingly, particularly in France, Germany, Italy, and Holland.

About 1960, Dr. Robert Egan in Houston presented his variation in technique of X-ray examination of the breast, which aroused keen interest on the part of the Cancer Control Program of the National Institutes of Health. His technique proved to be reproducible by others, who found that they also could achieve an acceptable accuracy of interpretation quickly. A dozen centers were soon established for indoctrination of radiologists, and mammography was launched on its career as a useful method in the diagnosis of breast diseases.

If we think about these facts a bit, an obvious remedy suggests itself. Why not have women examined when they are apparently well, before they find lumps, examine them with palpation (feeling) and the X ray, and ferret out the cancers at an earlier stage? Then we might ask: If we did find cancers in an earlier stage, would it make a real difference in how long a woman would live? Could she really be cured if the cancer were found earlier? And if this were so, how much would mammography contribute to the final results?

The author, a radiologist, early saw the potential of this "old-new" technique, and was in charge of one of the training centers located in New York City. The first mammogram, or X ray of the breast, seen by the author in Dr. Egan's laboratory at the University of Texas M. D. Anderson Hospital and Tumor Institute in Houston, was of a breast cancer which could not be felt at the time of operation but which had been discovered at the X-ray examination. The concept that herein lay a method for detection of breast cancer in a prepalpable stage took root and blossomed into the next phase of the story— a screening program in which women at random would be examined for breast cancer with the hope that earlier diagnosis might lead to a reduction in the mortality rate from this disease.

But first let's consider what is meant by "screening." By way of illustration, suppose you have a plastic bag filled with sand. Interspersed with the sand are pebbles of sizes and shapes varying from very tiny to very large, some round and some irregular. If you feel the bag quickly, you can probably pick out the fairly large pebbles. If you are more careful, you can probably detect some of the smaller ones. But you will probably miss the very small ones. If you now pour the sand through sieves with smaller and smaller holes, you will catch more and more of the smaller pebbles. If you vary the type of hole in the sieve, you may pick up irregular stones as well as smooth round ones.

Screening is really like using sieves to detect abnormalities. In the breast, most abnormal lumps can be found by palpation. Some lumps can be found only by the shadow they produce on an X ray. Some are too small to be detected by any of our present techniques. These may show up a few months later when they have grown large enough for our finest sieves. The screening process also presupposes that we are examining women who have not detected anything wrong with their own breasts and are coming in for just a checkup. Of course, it is at such times that the screening process will be more likely to find abnormalities in their earliest stages when they are most amenable to treatment and cure.

In 1963 a carefully conducted statistical study was begun by the Health Insurance Plan (HIP) of Greater New York under contract with the National Institutes of Health. The study, initiated by the author, was supervised by Sam Shapiro, vice-president of the Health Insurance Plan and in charge of research and statistics, and by the late Dr. Michael B. Shimkin, then associate director of the National Cancer Institute, with the invaluable assistance of Wanda Venet, R.N., and Dr. Louis Venet.

The Health Insurance Plan is a prepaid subscriber plan that offers comprehensive medical care through thirty-one medical groups located in Greater New York. For the study, 62,000 women were chosen from twenty-three of the groups to participate in the program. These women, aged forty to sixty-four, were chosen at random as 31,000 carefully matched pairs. In this way 31,000 women were then designated as the control group, while their counterparts constituted the study group.

Women in the control group received their usual medical care when they applied for it. Over the years, many of them developed breast symptoms and visited their group physicians for care. Some required breast operations, and occasional cancers were found and treated. The 31,000 women of the study group, on the other hand, were invited to come in for an extensive interview for data that might be helpful in future studies, a clinical examination, usually by a surgeon of the group, and mammography or X-ray study of the breasts. The examination was repeated each year for three years. After the third annual examination, no further studies were made. Enough time has now elapsed for statistical comparison of the two groups of women.

The results of an eighteen-year follow-up of all women showed a remarkable reduction in the number of deaths from breast cancer in the study group as compared with those in the control. About 25 percent fewer women of all ages died of breast cancer in the study group than in the control group. Treatment in both groups was the same. The characteristics of the women—age, number of children, family history, etc. —were the same. The only difference was the periodic breast examination, which included mammography. This difference accounted for a remarkable saving of lives. One could say that if the control-group women had been exposed to the same examination, perhaps one third of those who have died would still be alive today. These are striking statistics.

Furthermore, when we evaluated the specific role of mammography, there were some startling conclusions. The clinical and the X-ray examinations were done independently so that neither clinician nor radiologist knew of the findings of the other. In this way, one could know which method led to the cancer diagnosis.

It is a known fact that in regular medical practice, when a breast cancer is suspected on clinical examination and the patient is referred to a radiologist for an opinion on mammography, both physicians will agree on the diagnosis in over 80 percent of proven cases. Only occasionally is a cancer suspected on the basis of X-ray findings without some abnormality on palpation. It is also unusual for a cancer to be obvious to the clinician and not apparent to the radiologist.

Much to the surprise of everyone, one-third of the cancers found in the Health Insurance Plan study were not felt by the expert clinician. At the same time, two-fifths of the cancers were noted by the surgeon but not detected by the radiologist. In only one-fifth of the cases were the cancers found by both physicians. More important, in the control group, fewer than one-half of the cancers were found on operation to be localized to the breast and without spread to the armpit glands, while in the study group, three-quarters of the cancers were localized to the breast.

The most striking fact to come out of the study is that out of forty-four cancers found only by mammography and not felt by the clinician, only one woman died in an eight-year period of follow-up. A final eighteen-year follow-up of the study shows about a 25-percent saving of lives from breast cancer in women who were examined as compared with those who were not. A recent Swedish study designed to check on the results of the Health Insurance Plan study has come up with a similar reduction in the death rate through mass screening. It should be emphasized that one-third of the women in the study group never had even one examination but have been included for statistical reasons. Also, only about one-third of the women who were actually examined had all four studies. Had all the women in the study group had all four examinations, more cancers would have been detected in an early stage and more lives probably saved.

The study, therefore, has proven that persuading women to undergo examination, which includes palpation and mammography, can save a substantial proportion of those with breast cancer. It also has told us that an examination must include not only the usual clinical examination (palpation), but also the X-ray study, and that the absence of even one of these methods results in the missing of many cancers in the earliest stages when treatment is most likely to be successful.

The author, however, was not satisfied. The techniques used in the HIP study were too time-consuming, too expensive, and too tiring to the patient and technician alike. He also felt that since well women were being examined repeatedly, the radiation dosage used should be reduced to very minimal, altogether safe levels.

This information led to the creation of the Stella and Charles Guttman Breast Diagnostic Institute in New

York City in 1968. Initiated with funds from Charles Guttman, a New York City philanthropist with a lifelong interest in helping his fellowman, especially in the medical field, the organization has operated in close association with the American Cancer Society, New York City division. The author, who is now medical director emeritus of the Institute, collaborated closely with Mr. Salvator Cicetti, executive director of the American Cancer Society, New York City division, to devise an efficient, accurate, economical, and safe method to include all important procedures for a thorough breast examination. Also, steps were taken to train paramedical personnel to assist physicians in the screening process. Various avenues have been explored to stimulate women at risk of breast cancer to accept and even seek breast examinations when they have no symptoms. Such measures are especially necessary in low-income groups. Similar techniques have been followed at the Strax Institute in Florida.

The Institute has received financial support from the American Cancer Society, the National Cancer Institute, several foundations including the Stella and Charles Guttman Foundation, the Bruner Foundation, the William G. Connell Foundation, and the Damon Runyon Memorial Fund, as well as the U.O.T.S., the Cancer 18 Group, and many private individuals. Initially, no charge was made for the Institute's screening services, which were available to all women living in New York City. The screening process includes a medical history, a clinical examination, and mammography (the use of thermography has been discontinued due to its questionable value). A description of these examinations will be found later in this book.

Particularly gratifying was the success of the Guttman

Institute in developing a practical method for earlier breast-cancer detection, and the impact this has had on the national scene. The American Cancer Society, which initiated the idea of multiple screening centers in the United States, was joined in 1973 by the National Cancer Institute in developing and funding a network of twenty-seven demonstration projects involving twenty-nine institutions throughout the United States to determine whether mass screening for breast cancer was practical. Each project agreed to screen at least 10,000 women a year, for five years, using the methods of clinical examination, mammography, and thermography. Emphasis was placed on the use of volunteers and staff of divisions and units of the American Cancer Society to encourage all women in the community to have this thorough examination.

Obviously, a mechanism had been developed to tell all women that methods for saving lives from breast cancer are available and that women owe it to themselves and their families to take advantage of this new hope.

In New York City today 50,000 women receive the complete examination every year at the Guttman Institute. A similar satellite center in Lauderhill, Florida, The Strax Institute, examines about 30,000 women every year. Today a minimal charge is made to partially defray expenses.

3

WHO IS MOST LIKELY TO DEVELOP BREAST CANCER?

Of every ten girl babies born in the United States, nine will never develop breast cancer. If we had a way of pinpointing the single female who will get breast cancer, we could concentrate our efforts on her.

Perhaps someday there will be a blood test, a urine test, or a combination of tests that will warn a physician: "You'd better watch this young woman. She is more likely to develop breast cancer than other women. Watch her closely to find the cancer in its earliest stage."

As of now, such reliable tests do not exist, although a great deal of research is being done.

It would also be immensely helpful if we had a test that would assure a woman that she had little or no chance of developing cancer. Since the nine out of ten women who will never develop breast cancer are likely to have *some* breast symptoms or signs—lumps, nipple discharge— an accurate test that would spare them and their physicians undue worry or alarm would be a real advance.

In the hope of developing meaningful tests, researchers have been collecting information for years about women with various types of breast problems. Today we have a few indicators which tell us that in certain situations the risk of developing breast cancer is greater. These situations are not sufficiently definite, however, to allow us to predict cancer in any individual woman, so all women must be on their guard.

Every physician is at least in part a sleuth. He ferrets out clues from what the patient tells him, from what he finds on physical examination, from reports on X-ray and laboratory examinations; he relates these to each other and comes up with a good guess as to what is wrong with his patient. This guess is what we call a *diagnosis*. Sometimes a diagnosis can be more a suspicion than a certainty. But the more careful the physician is and the greater his acumen, the more often he will make an accurate diagnosis.

Today the physician working with clinical clues is only part of a larger medical team. Assisting him are a number of highly skilled investigators who bring knowledge from various new medical specialties. In the field of breast cancer, one of the most interesting of this highly skilled new breed is the epidemiologist.

These researchers try to discover clues from the environment, both inside and outside a human being, that can lead to solutions of medical problems. Just as the clinician seeks clues in his individual patient, the epidemiologist looks for telltale signals in large populations. These signals may be local, national, or international. They may be clues in the physical environment, in the types of food eaten by various human groups, in the genetic makeup of specific people, or in differences in blood types. The concept of epidemiology is universal. It deals in statistics and percentages and attempts to relate facts to each other. A recent discovery of this science was the association of cigarette smoking and lung cancer, which has now been generally accepted by the medical community. But even when the evidence is not complete, it often gives direction to future research.

For many years breast cancer has occupied the attention of these supersleuths. The challenge of a deadly illness that affects so many women, and that has so many interesting coincidences, has been great. Small wonder that some of the world's keenest minds have focused on the problem of breast cancer. Progress has been made, although the entire answer still eludes us. What does the epidemiologist tell us about breast cancer?

The most striking aspect of this disease is that it is gender-related. Even though men also have nipples and breast tissue, breast cancer is one hundred times more common in women than in men. Being a male affords a tremendous protection against the disease. The few men who do contract it usually do so at an older age—late in the fifties or sixties—and the breasts of these men sometimes show signs of development toward the female type.

Age, too, plays a most important role. Breast cancer is primarily a disease of mature women. It is quite unusual in women under the age of thirty, although it does occur. Only very rarely do young girls develop breast cancer.

When they do, it is of an entirely different type from that seen in adult women. It occurs so infrequently in young women that the chances are very great that a lump, even an obvious one, in a girl under twenty-five is due to a benign condition and not a cancer. For reasons that are not altogether clear, breast cancer begins to make its appearance usually after the age of forty. As a woman grows older, her chances of contracting it become greater. The increase continues through life, so that at age seventy a woman is many times more likely to develop breast cancer than at age forty.

This relationship to age is striking in the United States, in northern Europe, and in Israel, but the epidemiologist tells us that it does not hold true throughout the world. In South America or Africa, the increase in incidence related to age stops at about age fifty and levels off. In Asia the curve actually dips downward, frequency of breast cancer at older ages being less than that under age fifty. Why this variation with age exists in different areas is not known.

Even more striking is the correlation of the occurrence of breast cancer with different parts of the world. Breast cancer is most common in Scandinavian countries (with the exception of Finland), the British Isles, the United States, Canada, and in Israel among Israeli women of northern European origin. It is least common in the Orient and Africa, where breast cancer is only a fifth or a sixth as frequent as in the United States, although breast-cancer rates are increasing in these areas. Southern Europe and South America have intermediate incidence rates. Interestingly, the place where a woman lives may be more important than where she comes from. First-generation Japanese women in Hawaii, for instance, develop cancer at about the same rate as do those in Japan. Their granddaughters, however, have incidence rates approaching those in the mainland United States.

There are even significant differences among various parts of the United States. Considerably fewer women in Hawaii and Alaska develop breast cancer than do women in other parts of the United States, and Eskimos have incidence rates similar to those in the Orient. But even among the other states, considerable differences exist: New York State tops the list, but a high risk of breast cancer extends throughout the northeastern part of the United States. Women in southern states have less breast cancer, Mississippi, for example, having about half the incidence of New York. The other areas of the country are intermediate in risk.

In New York City, where statistics for ethnic groups are collected, black women have been found to develop breast cancer less frequently than white women. Puerto Rican women are affected even less frequently. Economic status also plays a part, with women in the upper income brackets having a higher frequency of breast cancer. Jewish women, who have a much lower incidence of cancer of the cervix (neck of the womb), have a greater risk of developing breast cancer than non-Jewish women. Jewish women born in the United States seem to incur a higher risk than their mothers who were born even in high-risk areas of Europe. Native American Jewish women in upper economic brackets have a 30-percent higher propensity for breast cancer than their non-Jewish neighbors. Why all this should be so is still a mystery.

Studies of large groups of women in different parts of the world have uncovered other interesting correlations. A woman who has her first full-term baby before the age of twenty has her risk of developing breast cancer reduced by two-thirds, and this protective effect persists through life, regardless of whether she has other children and at whatever ages she may have had them.

The protective effect applies only to a full-term birth. A first full-term birth when the mother is past thirty seems to increase the risk of breast cancer.

The number of children a woman bears also seems to be relevant. Women who have not had any full-term births have the greatest chance of developing breast cancer—in fact, such a woman incurs two to three times the risk of a woman with three children.

The ovaries are important in this connection. Women who, for whatever reason, lose their ovaries when they are under the age of 35 seldom get breast cancer.

An interesting relationship exists between frequency of breast cancer and the age at onset of menstruation and the age at menopause. In general, the more years of menstrual activity, the greater the likelihood for breast cancer to develop. Early onset of periods and late menopause carry with them an increased risk by a factor of about two.

It used to be thought that women who nursed their children were protected from breast cancer. Recent worldwide data contradict this concept. Nursing or not nursing appears to have no effect on the incidence of breast cancer.

Family history has also been found to be an important risk factor. There are well-authenticated records of "cancer families" in which the frequency of cancer is especially high. This also applies to breast cancer. There are, indeed, families in which several sisters, mother, and several aunts all have developed breast cancer. All women in such families need careful observation all their lives. Generally speaking, daughters of women who have had breast cancer have an increased tendency toward the disease, particularly if the mother had breast cancer before her change of life. It should be emphasized that by far the largest number of women with breast cancer have daughters who *never* develop the same disease.

Outside of the rare "cancer family," the inherited tendency to breast cancer presents only a slightly increased hazard. It means only that if a woman has a mother or sister who developed breast cancer before her menopause, her chances of developing the disease are increased from her usual odds of 1 in 10 to 1 in 5. The chances still are 5 to 1 that she will never develop the disease. However, she should have periodic breast examinations using the best methods available in her community.

All in all, the preponderance of evidence points to some part of "femaleness" as being deeply involved in the initiation or promotion of breast cancer. This has led to an ongoing study of the hormone balance in women and the differences in their production of the various hormones. There is a real possibility that a blood or urine test might be developed that could help identify women at higher risk.

Up to now, we have been describing risk factors found in the history provided by the woman. In the course of a complete breast examination, other hints may be noted. Some of these require more study before they can be properly evaluated. Some are already showing signs of being perhaps the markers we are all looking for—those data that can identify the woman who has to be watched more carefully because she has a greater risk of developing breast cancer.

Thus, on clinical examination, some experts feel strongly that well-defined masses that turn out to be benign cysts containing fluid—clear or cloudy or tinged with color—may be associated with breasts that have a greater risk for developing cancer than breasts that do not have these large cysts. Many others do not agree with these conclusions. Part of the difficulty is that many physicians have become accustomed to such technical terms as "fibrocystic disease" or "fibromastitis" or just "cystic" to describe the nodular character of a breast which in many cases feels like a multitude of small lumps. Practically every woman whose breasts have been examined by a physician has been told at one time or another that she has some type of "cysts" or "cystic disease." The woman concludes that she has some sort of disease or at least a condition that may lead to trouble. The truth is that probably all women have cysts—tiny ones—that could be seen microscopically, but that this is a normal though constantly changing condition that calls for no concern whatsoever. The only possible relationship of cysts with increased risk of breast cancer refers to the very large cysts that are occasionally detected and are easily remedied with aspiration (drawing the fluid out with a small needle). Such women should be more certain to examine their breasts *regularly* and to have a complete breast examination periodically.

Mammography, or X-ray examination of the breasts—about which we shall have more to say later—can also show up details of breast structure that seem to be related to increased risk of developing breast cancer. In such cases, another mammogram in two or three months may be necessary. Observation in such instances is most likely perfectly safe. In other cases some investigators think there is a relationship between certain patterns of the milk ducts on the mammograms or the enlargement of veins that suggests potential trouble. The radiologist will report that, although no evidence of cancer as such is present, there is sufficient suspicion to warrant an early restudy.

Thermography—the heat pattern of the breast—may also be an indicator of increased risk. In some 15 to 20 percent of women, increased heat is detected in one breast when all other examinations are normal. Such breasts are considered by some to be at increased risk and should be watched more carefully and examined more frequently than others. Whether concern about the increased heat is really necessary will be proved only after many more studies are concluded. At the present time, not enough data are available to consider thermography of sufficient value to counteract the additional expense of the examination. Modern improvements in technique in mammography seem to make thermography less important as a screening agent.

Another facet of the problem of increased risk, the one that is probably the least understood of all, refers to psychological factors that might have to do with initiating the disease, or with laying the groundwork in the emotional and glandular makeup that might place the woman at increased risk. Such concepts have been broached over the years by psychiatrists in Europe, a radiologist in France, and psychologists in San Francisco, where some work in this direction has been attempted. The hope is that such thoughts may lead to a questionnaire which could identify a high-risk group of women. Such studies are still in the embryonic stage, however. There is no conclusive proof at this time that anxiety, emotional states, or psychological conditions are important in the development of breast cancer. A study to shed light on this problem is under way at the Guttman and Strax institutes under the auspices of psychiatrists at Memorial Hospital in New York City.

Many factors associated with increased chances of developing breast cancer have been mentioned. Most of these factors concern only small changes in risk. But combinations of factors increase such risk changes substantially and may be helpful in deciding that some women should be examined more often or more thoroughly than others. Women who recognize themselves in some of the groups we have mentioned above should not be alarmed, because we are dealing only with small increases in chances of developing breast cancer. However, these women should definitely take advantage of our recent findings on earlier detection. Intensive study of risk factors by the outstanding statisticians of the American Cancer Society, Seidman and Garfinkel, have led to the conclusion that only about 25 percent of women who developed cancer have any of the known risk factors and that we have to consider all women over thirty-five as at risk of having or developing the disease.

As yet we cannot tell in advance which women will develop the disease. We do not know why it is that of two women who are almost exactly the same age, height, and weight, with a similar menstrual history, who have had the same number of children and have perhaps nursed them the same length of time, one should suddenly find herself with breast cancer while the other goes through life without the slightest breast trouble.

In all such clue-hunting we must be careful not to jump to hasty conclusions which turn out to be fancy rather than fact. Let us not be like the professor who spent many years studying the life of the flea and for his final great experiment gathered together a quantity of the little fellows. Gently, he took one out of the jar, placed it before him, and said, "Fly, flea!" and the flea flew away. He repeated the experiment three times with the same result. He then placed a fourth flea in front of him, removed its wings and said, "Fly, flea!" but nothing happened. "When you remove the wings of a flea," he concluded, "it becomes deaf!"

And lest you think this story has taught you the lesson of not jumping to conclusions, it should be pointed out that fleas do not have wings at all and can only jump, not fly!

4

WHAT WE KNOW ABOUT THE BREAST

The female 100-foot whale cavorting in far-off ocean depths, the sure-footed female mountain goat nimbly jumping from crag to crag atop a high mountain, the 12-foot-high, two-ton elephant cow trudging along on Africa's savanna, and the tiny, blind female mole burrowing under your lawn—all share an important trait with you. They are all mammals and as such carry the badge of their ancestral common bond with you—they have mammary glands, or breasts. They give birth to living young in various stages of immaturity. The breasts are there to supply the proper nourishment when life struggles to start.

What is this remarkable structure, how does it develop, and what do we know about how it is affected by the environment around us and by other parts of the body, especially the hormones from the endocrine glands?

When our first ancestral mammal mother gave birth to her first live young, both found that nature had provided well. A remarkable transformation had been taking place while the fetus was developing in its mother. A series of sweat glands of the skin on either side of the abdomen had undergone a change and been turned into an apparatus for the production of milk—a new complete substance with just the right ingredients to maintain life and nourish the infant.

In the sixth week of development of the human fetus in the womb, a mammary ridge can be detected, with an elevation of skin running along each side of the chest and abdomen and extending from the armpits to the groin. Skin sweat glands along this ridge develop into rudimentary milk-bearing structures—the breasts, similar to the situation that exists in other mammals. The number and location of these mammary glands or teats or breasts depends on the needs of the particular mammal—the number of young in the litter and the convenience for suckling or nursing. In the human, one breast develops on each side of the chest. Occasionally, evidence of our ancestry is disclosed by the presence of a rudimentary breast or nipple elsewhere along the milk line. Sometimes a well-developed extra breast or nipple or both may be present. They are no cause for concern and may be removed for cosmetic reasons if desired.

The breast is a complex, highly specialized structure that produces a fluid called milk, which contains the proper proportion of food elements for a human infant.

This nutriment is contained in a vessel specially shaped and located for the convenience of both mother and infant.

The breast is made up of three types of tissue: the delicate glandular component in which milk is actually formed; the intricate branching duct system that brings the milk to the surface at the nipple; and the supporting tissue. The latter is made of a firm substance, called fibrous tissue, and fat.

The glandular system is made up of a myriad of microscopic cells which can remove substances from the blood and turn them into milk. These tiny glands, or *acini*, open into microscopic ducts which lead to larger and larger ductules until they empty eventually into the main ducts (which may vary from six to fifteen) with openings in the nipple. The entire breast is enclosed for support in a strong elastic envelope which is an extension of the covering of those chest muscles called the pectoralis major and minor. The firmness of this envelope gives the breast its protuberant appearance. When it becomes lax with age or after many childbirths, the breast sags.

It is particularly important to remember that the breast extends well up into the armpit and over to the breastbone. A thorough examination of the breast must include these areas as well as the obvious portion. There is a variable amount of fat and of the tougher fibrous tissue within the breast which supports and protects the delicate structures. The amount of fat in the breast varies with the general body build.

The breast has a liberal supply of blood vessels, nerves, and lymphatic vessels. Its physiological changes are very closely associated with the glandular or endocrine system of the body. Throughout the lifetime of a woman the breast—its size, its structure, and its function—is carefully regulated by such glands as the pituitary, ovaries, adrenals, and thyroid. The breast is certainly not in a static condition. It undergoes constant dynamic changes—changes that are sometimes associated with harmless breast conditions, sometimes with cancer. Many arteries and their branches bring the necessary oxygen and nutrition for breast function, and many veins are present to remove waste products.

The lymphatic system is very important. There are small lymph channels in the breast which drain the breast substance as well as the overlying skin. The lymph ducts contain a fluid called lymph, which in turn contains products of metabolism of the glandular system and other structures. The lymph system is an additional mechanism for removing waste material from the factory that is producing milk products. There are dozens of way stations or lymph nodes (sometimes called glands) in this network of lymph channels. A few are present in the breast substance, many more are located in the armpit, some can be found under the breastbone, and some above the collarbone (the supraclavicular region). These nodes are intimately connected with the spread of breast cancer. They contain highly specialized cells called lymphocytes which stop, attack, and destroy breast-cancer cells. The lymph nodes act as a front-line defense to prvent the cancer cells from overrunning the body. It is true that some cancer cells penetrate blood vessels and in this way wander off to outlying parts of the body. In these situations, other defenses present in the blood come into play. Cancer cells attempt to overwhelm the defense mechanism of the lymph nodes. Most of the defense is centered in the lymph nodes of the armpit. Because breast cancer too often involves these nodes, the treatment of breast cancer has been devised to remove and examine these nodes. Such investigation of the axilla can be done most thoroughly only by removal of the pectoralis (chest) muscles, which run from the chest to the upper arm. Therefore, surgical procedures commonly remove all or some of those structures in the course of the operation for breast cancer.

DEVELOPMENT

In infancy and childhood, both male and female have tiny breasts which are made up of a few dilated ducts and fibrous tissue with a minimal rudimentary glandular system. Occasionally as a result of the effect of the mother's hormones, a breast discharge may be present in the infant—so-called witches' milk—which is of no consequence and disappears shortly. After puberty, the female breast develops and becomes larger and firmer. With maturity, the glandular system develops and lobules or small glands form in which milk is produced. In the male, none of this glandular-system development usually occurs. However, at puberty one or both breasts may enlarge temporarily. This is of no clinical importance.

Very definite changes occur during the menstrual cycle. After menstruation, the endocrine system starts to prepare the breast for possible pregnancy. The egg is released in midcycle. At that time the breast is increasing in size and becoming more tender because the glandular system is developing and the breast is swollen with extra fluid. This accounts for the common premenstrual discomfort in the breasts. If pregnancy does not occur, the swelling disappears and the breast returns to its resting state. If pregnancy does occur, the glandular system continues to develop, more lobules and acini are produced, the duct system proliferates to keep pace, and the fibrous tissue and fat also develop. In short, the breast continues to enlarge, becomes firmer, and is eventually filled with the proper machinery for milk production.

If a mother nurses her child, the breast continues to be efficient and the supply of milk is continuous. If nursing is not instituted, the breast gradually changes back to its normal resting state. After every childbearing, however, the breast usually remains larger than it was before the pregnancy, because there is more fat and less glandular substance.

After the menopause, profound changes occur in the breast. The breast usually becomes larger because of an increase in the amount of fat, and "involution" or disappearance of glandular substance takes place. Most breasts after the menopause appear superficially to be substantial glandular organs, but they are primarily reservoirs of fat.

The changes described are initiated and promoted by hormones mostly from the ovaries, the pituitary, and the adrenal glands. Disturbances in the hormone glands are reflected in abnormalities of the breasts. If there is ovarian disturbance in a young woman with menstrual abnormalities, the breast may seem normal in appearance but will lack development of glandular substance and be composed mostly of fat, so that a twenty-year-old woman may have the same breast as a seventy-year-old. On the other hand, a seventy-year-old woman who still has ovarian secretion, or sufficient adrenal hormones to make up an ovarian deficiency, may have young-looking breasts. Whether such unusual development may protect or predispose to breast cancer is not known, but offers a fruitful field for study.

HARMLESS BREAST CONDITIONS

There is a remarkable variation in breasts. They may be very small, resembling those of males, or truly enormous. They may be firm or full or sagging. The nipples may be flat, inverted, small, or large and erect. The areola (the dark area around the nipple) may be dark brown and large or small and pale pink. The breast may be very lumpy, with thousands of small nodules, or be completely free of lumpiness. The breasts may be extremely tender all over or only in limited areas, or they may be insensitive to the touch. They may produce a dragging feeling constantly or only at certain times during the month. These sensations may be relieved by special bras, diuretics, or certain vitamins. One breast may be substantially larger or more sensitive than the other.

Yet all may be completely normal breasts and may never develop any serious condition. As a matter of fact, most, if not all, women have sufficient breast symptoms at one time or another to cause anxiety and warrant a visit to a physician. Such examinations are important and should be sought for the slightest reason. The reassurance of a normal examination is often vital to the well-being of a woman.

Considering that there are so many normal variations, it is difficult to spell out what breast conditions warrant special observation. Apart from obvious things, such as infection or abscesses, one could say that a normal breast is one that does not have cancer. After all, it is only cancer that physicians and women are concerned about. The physician has labels for various harmless or benign breast conditions, but as long as they have no relationship to cancer, they should remain just labels. For the sake of completeness and because many women hear about such labels (which carry the connotation of disease), let's look at some of these benign conditions more closely.

Fibrocystic Disease

This is often called "fibrocystic mastopathy" or "cystic disease," or the woman is just told that she is "cystic." It is the most common cause of a lump in a woman aged thirty to fifty. The only importance of this condition is that it often is associated with lumps or a lump, painful or not, and that operations are performed to find out the nature of the lump. About half of all operations on the female breast are performed for fibrocystic disease. If we knew in advance that the lump felt by physician, woman, or both was not a cancer, an operation would not be needed. Unfortunately, we still cannot be absolutely certain about such lumps, and a biopsy, or removal of a small portion to examine under the microscope, is a must to make sure that all is well.

Nevertheless, with the addition of mammography (X-ray examination of the breast), some of these lumps can be recognized as large cysts—harmless collections of fluid which can be drained by the surgeon using a thin needle. Most surgeons aspirate localized masses when possible, but if no fluid is obtained, biopsy becomes essential. In most women these large cysts (which can recur many times and be multiple) disappear after the menopause.

Most pathologists—those physicians who are expert at diagnosing tissues under a microscope—agree that 90 percent or more of the specimens they examine contain evidence of "fibrocystic disease." Accordingly, it is not a disease but a normal variation. It is also generally agreed that there probably is no connection between the usual fibrocystic changes and cancer, although many cancerous breasts will also have this condition. An infrequent fibrocystic change, seen only under the microscope and called *epithelial hyperplasia*, may have some connection with cancer change.

The important part of the story is that a woman who is told she has fibrocystic disease should not be unduly alarmed. It's usually just another way for her physician to tell her that he is quite sure she has no serious condition, but that she has more or less lumpy breasts—which are very common—and that she should continue to be examined regularly. The term "normal" when applied to breasts covers wide variations, and the concern of the average physician that he might be missing a cancer in any individual patient is so great that he tends to put a label on the woman. Many physicians do not agree on what fibrocystic disease means, although many use the technical term. Physicians set up guidelines for themselves on what is "normal" so that they can say to a woman, "I find no evidence of cancer. You have a variation commonly found in normal breasts. Please continue to examine your own breasts regularly and report to me promptly if you feel anything unusual. Otherwise, your best insurance is to have a complete breast examination once a year. I will now teach you the technique of breast self-examination so that you will know what is normal for you."

Fibroadenoma

This is a solid lump most commonly seen in women in their teens or twenties. The lumps are smooth, regular, and usually single, although more than one may be present in one or both breasts. They are usually not tender. Fibroadenomas contain normal breast elements surrounded by an envelope or capsule. Since they are definite lumps, they can frighten a young woman. It is extremely rare for a fibroadenoma to become malignant. The only two problems connected with this condition are that it exists not only in the breast but in the mind of its possessor, and that occasionally it may grow during changes associated with pregnancy. Again, if we were absolutely certain that a definite lump was not cancer, it could be left alone. For the reasons mentioned, however, most physicians advise removal of such lumps. Removal is often an extremely simple procedure that will confirm the diagnosis and eliminate a source of tension.

Papilloma

Nipple discharge is a worrisome condition. The woman who is so affected becomes quite disturbed. Only rarely is the usual non-bloody discharge associated with cancer, unless there are other changes. As a rule, the discharge is caused by irritation within ducts and does not mean that a cancer is brewing. Such a woman deserves, of course, regular periodic checkups.

Occasionally, a discharge is bloodstained or bloody.

The bloodstained drop is often associated with a benign papilloma, a small harmless growth in a duct usually near the nipple. Such a growth is best removed; the operation is simple and in only a very small proportion of patients is it associated with an early cancer. An unusual clear yellow discharge also requires special attention. If the discharge is associated with a mass, it arouses more concern. The discharge that is profuse and bloody requires closer attention because it may be associated with a cancer. The fluid is usually studied for its cell content for a more definite diagnosis.

Hematoma (sometimes called *Fat Necrosis*)

Because of the breast's location, it is readily subject to injury. Occasionally injury may produce bleeding beneath the skin which appears as a discolored area in the skin (black-and-blue mark) and an associated mass under the skin. This is a frightening experience. It can be said, however, that there has never been an authenticated case of such an injury that has led to breast cancer. When breast cancer is present, an injury may call attention to a preexisting mass, but the injury has no relation to it. Of course, all masses should be under observation by a physician if he so decides, or until definitive treatment is begun. Mammography is most useful in following progress and in making sure no other condition is present.

Infections

The breast, like any organ, is subject to infection. A condition known as *mastitis* sometimes occurs during or immediately following pregnancy, and may be related to a cracked or injured nipple. An abscess may also develop in the breast, secondary to severe inflammation of the large ducts without any apparent cause. Such infections usually are treated successfully with compresses and antibiotics. Occasionally, surgery is needed for drainage.

Sometimes a superficial vein in the skin of the breast becomes inflamed (*thrombophlebitis* or "Mondor's disease"). This results in a painful thickened vein on the surface of the breast usually showing skin retraction. It may take several months to clear completely.

Another harmless condition is "Tietze's disease," an irritation of the cartilage portion of one or two ribs near the breastbone. Because it is noticed in the general area of the inner portion of the breast, a woman may consider it a breast condition. It is important for her to remember that the condition is not related to the breast, and usually corrects itself in several weeks.

Extremely Small or Large Breasts

These conditions cause much anguish, but of course are within normal variations. Attempts to make small breasts larger by means of hormone injections are fraught with danger. However, plastic surgeons can insert an implant of a plastic envelope containing silicone with good results. Injections of silicone (not in an implant) are dangerous, and should be avoided.

Very large breasts can be treated only by a plastic operation, called mammoplasty, which usually is quite successful.

There are women who have had one or many—even seven or eight—operations to remove various benign lumps. In such cases, some plastic surgeons remove the breast tissue under the skin and replace it with silicone implants. Results are usually very acceptable.

Eczema of the Nipple

Irritations of the skin of the nipple or its surrounding area (the areola) may be due to clothing, cosmetics, or minor infections. The condition is called eczema of the nipple and is usually of no consequence. However, any such change which does not clear up completely in two to three weeks should be checked by a physician. It may be confused with a more important condition, called Paget's disease of the nipple, which is a form of cancer.

5

WHAT WE KNOW ABOUT BREAST CANCER

A prime characteristic of living things is change. Every living cell is in a constant state of flux from the moment of its birth. Thus, every organ of the body is different from one minute to the next, though the difference may be only microscopic.

These changes are produced by chemical messengers from various endocrine glands, such as the pituitary, ovary, adrenals, and thyroid, present in the environment of the cells which determine their nutrition and growth. They affect and modify the "programming" inherent in every cell that is based on the makeup of its genes. This vast, complex mechanism exists solely for the purpose of keeping the living organism in a state of balance with its external environment. A basic mechanism of this sort is present in all living things from the most primitive single-cell amoeba to humans themselves.

The delicate mechanism of the cell is subjected to constant strain and stress in its perilous journey through life. The outcome of this struggle depends on the power of destructive forces and the strength of the defensive mechanism.

One of the most insidious and mysterious of stresses to which humans as well as other living things are subjected is cancer. The secrets of its cause and how it performs its deadly work still elude us. Much research is being carried on in centers all over the world directed toward solving these mysteries, and it is the profound hope and expectation of all mankind that this work will lead to a complete understanding in the near future. As of this writing, however, all we have are hopes and a few very promising leads.

We can identify a breast-cancer cell under a microscope. An expert can look at a group of cells and determine with an extremely high degree of accuracy whether a cell in question is cancerous or not. This microscopic examination remains our best and most accurate method of making a true diagnosis. It is the basis for the biopsy, at which time some of the tissue in question is subjected to a microscopic examination. Though we do not know how a cancer cell originates, we do know a good deal about its behavior. We know, for instance, that such a cell behaves like a maverick. It no longer follows the rules set for orderly checks and balances. The computer of the cancer cell seems to be newly programmed. Some cancers continue to be controlled by glandular hormones and produce their harmful effects slowly. Others, however, even in the early stages, behave like completely independent operators with no respect for the rest of the organism; they grow wildly, and cause quick destruction.

The intricate mechanism that spells the change from a normal cell to a cancer cell is probably the same in all cancers, even though the promoting causes that start the change may be different. The effect, however, varies not only with cancers of different organs, but also with individual cancers of the same organ. A common misconception exists that "cancer is cancer" and that once cancer starts in the body, the individual is doomed. This is far from the truth. Hundreds of thousands of individuals have been cured of cancer.

There are broadly two groups of cancers, and we call them "primary" and "secondary." A primary cancer develops from the original cell transformation in an organ such as the breast or bowel or lung. As long as the cancer stays confined to its organ site, the damage it does is local—the part of the organ involved no longer maintains its usual function, but the effect on the rest of the body is only minimal. The great danger of cancer is that secondary cancers may develop. These secondary cancers (or *metastases*) are due to a spreading of the cancer cells from their original place to another organ where they may succeed in setting up new colonies. It is these secondary cancers that produce the destruction and cause the real damage we associate with the disease.

Some organs, like the breast, are frequently the site of primary cancers and seldom the site of secondary cancers. Some organs, like the liver, are only occasionally the site of a primary cancer, but are often involved with a secondary process. Some organs, like the lungs, are frequently the site of both.

It should be emphasized that an individual who is affected with—and cured of—a primary cancer does not usually develop another primary cancer in some other organ. "Cancer," as a disease, is highly organ-oriented. Thus, primary cancer of the breast is a disease unto itself that has nothing to do with primary cancer of the lung. This all means that if a breast cancer is detected and treated when it is confined to the breast, the woman is most likely cured. Of course, she must continue to have periodic thorough examinations, especially to safeguard the other, presumably healthy, breast.

Breast cancer occurs most often after the age of thirty-five. For a period of time which varies with different women, the cancer remains localized in the breast and the body defenses hold the upper hand. As cancer cells leave the main growth to wander from the breast, they are apparently destroyed. After a variable time, which may be several years, the protective mechanism becomes deficient and the wandering cells are able to survive and establish new colonies in other organs. These new growths then tend to destroy their new homes and lead to widespread disease. We do not yet know what viruses or hormone disturbances or dietary indiscretions stimulate dormant cancer cells to proliferate. Nor do we know why some cancer cells leave their local site and set off to carry their destructive influences elsewhere. Nor do we clearly know how the defensive mechanism works and why it does well for many years and then seemingly breaks down. Nor do we know why the breast is such a common site of cancer.

What we do know—and what is most important for

all women—is that if the cancer is detected in its early clinical stages, which means when it is truly localized to the breast and has not spread even to the local nodes, it is curable in a very high percentage of patients. The woman may then live out her life span as though she had never contracted the disease. In other words, breast cancer is a curable disease—not a fatal one—*if* it is detected when it is early and minimal.

6

WHAT CONSTITUTES A BREAST EXAMINATION

Mrs. B.C., thirty-four and the mother of five, reproached her family physician. "I have known you for fifteen years. For the past twelve years I have been visiting the gynecologist you referred me to on a regular basis. During all this time, neither you nor the gynecologist has examined my breasts, except for an occasional perfunctory examination when I was pregnant. Don't you think I have a legitimate complaint? I have heard recently that there are newer methods that are of great help in finding breast abnormalities. Shouldn't I get the benefit of the latest?''

This conversation is an example of the growing awareness on the part of women that their breasts—that part of their anatomy which is the focus of so much concern — deserve much greater interest from and observation by their physicians than has been the case heretofore. The breast is easily accessible to examination by the woman and the physician alike. The use of procedures in addition to palpation is increasing as more people become aware of their availability and usefulness.

What does a breast examination mean to the modern woman, or what should it mean?

There are two types of breast examination. Both are vital to the well-being of the woman, and both should be accepted by her as a duty to herself and to those dear to her, and as a right.

The first type, and very important, is breast self-examination. And the second is examination by others, primarily a physician using his hands and eyes, and allied health professionals using new technology to expand the horizon of detection.

Certainly the oldest, and by far the most common, method for earlier breast-cancer detection is BSE—breast self-examination by the woman herself. This procedure is the simplest to apply, the least expensive, the most readily available, and it improves in value with regular repetition. It can be used profitably at any age.

Many women, however, never have the inclination or the confidence to examine their own breasts. They seem to be turned off by the variations in consistency and the irregularities they find. Many of them actually complain that they develop anxieties when they feel their breasts because they suspect they have lumps. A woman needs to be aware that a breast is not a homogeneous mass, but that it normally contains various structures, some of which are felt as nodules, thickenings, or small lumps. She should be examined thoroughly with all our modern techniques to make sure that all is well before she is taught breast self-examination on a one-to-one basis on her own breasts. She can then be reassured that her breasts are normal even though there are little irregularities. Every woman's breast is different in this respect from all others. Besides, each breast varies in texture from year to year and often during even a single month. An intelligent woman's fingers are an excellent method of breast examination because every woman can become aware of her own breast makeup and can readily detect a change, often a very small one. The average woman can probably become as expert in examining her own breast as a general physician who sees her for the first time and has not had the benefit of repeated earlier examinations of that particular breast.

What is important, of course, is any *change* a woman finds from one examination to the other. Let's describe the actual technique of a breast examination. It's simple and easy to do.

The basic principles involved are that the examination should be started when the skin is wet and soapy, as during a shower or bath, and that the palmar (flat) surface of the fingers—not the tips—be used. The hands should be relaxed and the touch gentle, and all portions of the breast must be examined, including the nipple and those portions that extend high into the armpit and near the breastbone. Some experts suggest a rotary motion in feeling the breast, area by area; others suggest a gentle stroking feeling either up and down or across. It is best to repeat the examination both in the upright position and lying down in bed after the examination in the shower. The examination should be done once a month, preferably at the same time. For menstruating women, the end of the period, when the breasts are less sensitive, is an excellent time. For others, the first of the month is an easy date to remember.

It is remarkable how sensitive a woman's fingers can become. A simple, painless examination that takes only a few minutes can detect a very tiny lump. With awareness of the need for breast self-examination must go the assurance that only very occasionally is even an apparently new lump the sign of a serious growth. However, only a physician can decide whether a mass needs further attention. A woman owes it to herself not to delay but to contact her physician whenever and as soon as she finds what she thinks is a lump or thickening that was not there on her last examination.

It cannot be emphasized too strongly that a breast self-examination on a monthly basis is a must. Not only is it the most common method for detection of breast cancer in early stages when practiced regularly, but it is most important even when regular periodic study by the physician is made—including the various modern techniques which will be described. In every screening study, involving apparently well women, a few women will get a clean bill of health and then find a new lump within a year of such an examination. Some of these turn out to be small early cancers which were not detectable in the previous complete study. Every woman who is alert to the problem and fulfills her responsibility to herself must continue self-examination all her life. She must not skip monthly examinations because she sees her physician on an annual or semi-annual basis.

The technique of breast self-examination is learned

easily from the accompanying diagram. At the time of the physician's examination, the details of this test should be gone over with him or her. It is the doctor's responsibility to teach a woman self-examination with her own hands on her own breast. Many a woman's life has been saved by this simple, easily learned examination. Every woman, regardless of her age, must do it regularly once a month. Every woman must urge her physician to teach her this technique on her own body. A pamphlet alone is just not enough. The hands of an expert physician are extremely valuable in assessing a breast. So, too, is breast self-examination when the woman has been taught the technique and is highly sensitive to even minor changes in her breasts. But it is important to realize that the earliest stage of a cancer may be associated with no lumps that can be felt by either the physician or the woman. That is why there is insistence that women undergo a periodic complete examination to include mammography. This is the only method we have to detect a cancer that is not palpable even by the fingers of an expert clinician.

The woman must not rely solely on her periodic mammogram to detect changes, however. A cancer may take eight to ten years from its onset in a microscopic stage before it becomes detectable with even our finest methods. If a woman is skilled at breast self-examination, she may be able to detect a change in her breast between the time of her last negative exam and her next scheduled study. Such an "interval cancer"—one that shows itself in the interval between exams—is likely to be in an early stage.

Thus, it is vital that a woman protect herself in both ways—by monthly careful BSE, and by periodic clinical and X-ray exams.

Clinical examination—which means examination

Remember: (1) Skin of breast and hands should be wet and soapy. (2) Use flat part of fingers. (3) Stroke gently, with a rotary motion. (4) Be sure to palpate all parts of the breast, including the armpit fold and the underportion. (5) Examine the breasts in the upright position as well as when lying down.

with the eyes, hands, and fingers of the physician—involves feeling the breast for a lump or seeing the changes in the skin as the result of such a lump. The lump must be close to the surface or large enough to stand out from its surroundings. If the breast is small, a very small lump can be felt. If the breast is very large, even a large lump may be difficult to detect. Lying on a small pea is uncomfortable, but it takes a princess to feel that same pea under a mattress. Thus, cancers in their early stages, when they are small, may be completely undetectable by feeling with the hands if the small cancer is in a large breast. When we consider that a woman's breast usually becomes larger and more fatty as she gets older, especially after the menopause, and when we consider that breast cancers become more common at the same time, the problem becomes apparent. At the very time when our "feeling ability" needs to be better, the breasts are larger and the process becomes more difficult.

Another aspect of the problem is that perhaps one-third of all cancers produce changes in the milk ducts in the early stages, which do not show up as lumps at all. These changes eventually coalesce and congeal to form a lump that can be felt, but by then the cancer may already have spread beyond the breast. In the early stages, that same cancer may not be felt at time of examination or even at time of operation.

Now we know that a small cancer in a large, fatty breast and many changes due to cancer in the ducts before a lump develops can be detected by the X ray with a high degree of accuracy. In other words, the X-ray examination called mammography does detect many cancers before they can be felt.

However, just as the clinical examination has its drawbacks (not every cancer can be felt), so mammography has its shortcomings (not every cancer can be seen on an X-ray film). On palpation, a cancer, to be felt, must be present as a lump that stands out amid its surroundings. In mammography, a cancer must have telltale signs on the film to make possible a diagnosis. Both methods occasionally fail, but fortunately they complement each other. Together, they form a very accurate team for detection. A large breast made up mostly of fat, in which a cancer lump may be difficult to feel, is viewed with more confidence by the radiologist, because the fat of the large breast presents a dark background on which the cancer stands out as a white mass. In addition, the diffuse changes in the ducts which do not show as a lump stand out as striking white dots called *microcalcifications*, and thus betray their appearance at an early stage of the cancer. And the cancer that produces changes in breast tissue by distortion of breast strands—or *trabeculae*—and which does not produce a palpable lump until the reaction of the breast adds dense fibrous tissue, can be detected on the X ray by virtue of these distortions.

Eventually, of course, all the cancers become large, palpable, and obvious, and produce changes in skin and glands. Eventually, too, the cancers show up as dense lumps and cause changes in breast structure so that the diagnosis on the X ray is easy to make. In time, therefore, cancers are detectable both on clinical examination and on mammography. This is true of perhaps nine out of ten cancers that are brought to physicians today. In these cases the X ray is used to complement the clinical diagnosis of cancer and to make sure there is no unsuspected trouble in the opposite breast.

Mammography may also show the clinician that the

suspicious lump is merely a cyst that needs only needle aspiration of fluid. Indeed, this situation is generally the case today.

However, stress is being placed more and more by many authorities on the use of mammography in "screening" for breast cancer. Under such circumstances, a woman has a complete breast examination as outlined in this book at a time when she has no apparent disturbance—no lumps or thickenings. At this stage, the X-ray examination becomes particularly valuable in detecting a tumor which cannot be felt. Such a mass— if a cancer—is usually in an early, localized state and responsive to treatment. Only by screening can most breast cancer be found when it is in a curable stage.

Since X rays are used in mammography, the dose of radiation applied is of importance. In recent years there has been improvement of the equipment used in this study. Special devices with special X-ray tubes and filters, plus special films, have made it possible to produce superior X-ray studies with minimal amounts of X rays. In centers where large-scale screening is done, the dose of radiation to the breasts can be made so small that all authorities are agreed that no danger is present or will develop even if a woman's breasts are subjected to repeated periodic examinations over many years. Today an annual examination is recommended for the average woman—unless other factors, such as strong family history or multiple operations, warrant more frequent study.

The X-ray examination is usually performed with two views, one up and down ("cranio-caudad") and the other from side to side ("medio-lateral" or "oblique"). This permits practically all of the breast to be examined. The examination is painless, quick, and convenient. Ordinarily no injections are used. If a breast discharge is present and is bloody, an injection of contrasting material may be made in the ducts to reveal further details of the duct mechanism.

Mammography usually involves the use of film as the recording medium, as is usually true in X-ray examinations of other parts of the body. In recent years the technical aspects of the procedure have been subjected to change in many quarters in an attempt to improve the quality of the images produced, the ease, speed, and economy of the examination, and the amounts of X rays used. The net result has been an improved mammographic image yielding more information with much less effort on the part of the technician. The improvements have been essentially in three directions: improved X-ray equipment to produce enhanced quality of the pictures; new ways to display the image to increase accuracy of diagnosis; and lower radiation dose.

New equipment with new types of tubes was originally developed by Prof. Charles Gros in Strasbourg, which produced greater detail in the images and which in turn made interpretation easier and more accurate. New films have since been introduced which have made it possible to produce these excellent images with minute amounts of X rays, so that there need be no concern about periodic examinations, even over many years.

Another important part of a breast examination is the history, or the medical interview. Details of personal, menstrual, childbearing, breast, and family history are helpful in evaluating whether a woman is likely to develop cancer and whether more frequent examinations are needed. These data collected uniformly in many thousands of screening examinations, such as are being sponsored in the United States by the American Cancer Society and the National Cancer Institute, may provide valuable insights into the development of breast cancer. In some centers, other means for breast-cancer detection are in various stages of development. Ultrasound energy is being used as a potential detector of cancer. Transillumination, in which powerful but cool lights are used to look through the breast, is also being tried in some places to differentiate solid masses from cysts. Aspiration of masses, in which a small amount of tissue is removed with a needle, is an additional means for detecting a cancer quickly. It should be emphasized that a negative result with a needle aspiration of this type does not rule out the possibility of a cancer.

The technique of a thorough breast examination varies widely in quality as well as quantity among physicians in various countries and even in different regions of the same country. Physical examination depends on the experience of the physician. Some physicians never develop expertise because they seldom examine a woman's breast unless she has breast symptoms. And even then, the examination may be cursory, taking only a minute or two. Compare this with the thirty minutes it may take an expert in history-taking and in the complete examination.

It should be emphasized, however, that only mammography can detect the cancer that is not palpable. In screening of apparently well women, only palpation and mammography are useful. If, however, an abnormality is palpable, the other techniques mentioned may be useful for complete assessment of the problem.

In short, every woman is entitled to the very best and most complete periodic breast examination available to her in her community. Never must she lose sight, however, of the need to supplement the examination with a regular, monthly breast self-examination.

7

THE CASE FOR MASS SCREENING OF WOMEN

Thirty-five years ago, the lot of a physician interested in preventing breast cancer was much easier than it is today. The average breast cancer received by the pathologist was 4 to 5 cm. or more in diameter and was detected by the woman herself. After a period of delay —sometimes weeks or months of hoping the lump would go away and keeping the problem to herself—the woman would bring her breast condition to her primary-care physician or her gynecologist. After another delay of weeks or months, the mass would be delivered to the surgeon, who would proceed to definitive treatment,

59

which was usually a one-stage operation with removal of the entire breast and both chest muscles and a thorough dissection of the armpit. The surgeon was armed with a consent form permitting such a procedure in the event that a frozen section proved positive. However, in spite of extensive surgery, most women were dead or dying within ten and often within five years of their surgery. Occasionally, in the course of surgery for an adjacent benign lesion, a small lesion with negative nodes was found accidentally.

Today, after many controversies and advances in detection, diagnosis, and therapeutic approach, the situation has changed. No longer is talk of breast cancer taboo. No longer are women loath to discuss their situation with family friends or physician. The media are full of accounts, some alarming, of so-called proper approaches to the breast-cancer problem. Many differences of opinion have surfaced in the areas of detection, diagnosis, and treatment. Many women and even their physicians are prey to confusion, doubt, and anxiety in this matter.

As I hope to show in this book, there are very well-founded reasons to hope for better results in the future. We now have evidence that detection of a cancer in the early stage can result in a long-term survival rate sufficient to equate in practical terms with reduced mortality. Also, we now have at our disposal procedures that can detect early-stage cancers. The task ahead is to make these procedures available throughout the population, regardless of financial and geographical considerations, and to motivate women to present themselves for examination. Let us consider how this might be done.

WHY SHOULD WE DO MASS SCREENING?

The *definitive diagnosis* of breast cancer is made by the pathologist. The step before the diagnosis involves the clinician—an internist, gynecologist, or surgeon—who is faced with a more or less frightened woman who comes in complaining of a lump, a localized pain, or a nipple discharge. A *differential diagnosis* is called for, with the subsequent and sometimes difficult decision whether to explore the breast or to wait watchfully. The clinician uses all the resources available in the community, in addition to inspection and palpation, to gather the information on which to base the vital decision.

There is a step before the clinical one, however, and that is *detection* of an abnormality that will propel the woman into the stream of medical care preliminary to the differential diagnosis. That initial step may be a suspicion on the part of the woman herself that a problem may be present, as found by her on periodic or accidental breast self-examination; or it may arise from accidental detection of pathology by a physician in the course of an examination for a nonbreast condition. Unfortunately, this has been our approach to cancer detection up till now: We wait for a woman to find her own abnormality, or hope that a physician will have the expertise or will even bother to examine the breast when the patient's symptoms point elsewhere. Our results, in terms of saving lives of women from breast cancer, have not been as good as they might be. In more than half the cases, the breast cancer is detected at too late a stage to effect a cure. Overall, probably not more than 25 to 30 percent of women are alive and free of disease ten years after diagnosis. We need a better way.

Consider the following:

1. We do not know the cause of breast cancer, nor do we have any method for preventing the disease.
2. We do not as yet have any combination of therapies, whether surgery, radiotherapy, or chemotherapy, that can cure the disease regardless of the stage at which it is diagnosed. We do not have the "magic bullet." We cannot cure metastatic disease.
3. The need for a real cure of the disease has never been greater. It is a serious problem of women, especially in the Western world, perhaps their most serious health problem. In this country, there has been an increasing incidence of the disease, so that today one in ten is afflicted, with a particularly steep rise in women under the age of fifty. And most important, the death rate from the disease in this country has been stationary for the past forty years.

When we consider what can be done about this problem, we must note the following:

1. It is general knowledge that detection of breast cancer in a localized stage with negative nodes leads today to an over-85-percent five-year survival rate. When nodes are involved, the survival rate drops to 53 percent or less. This is still the stage at which the majority of breast cancers are detected.
2. An important reason for this poor showing may be that over 90 percent of breast cancer is first detected by women themselves, who then bring the problem to their physicians. It seems obvious that, since most

breast cancer today is not localized when first seen by the clinician, a means must be found to have women present themselves for examination when the disease is at an earlier stage than is commonly the case. This means, in a practical way, detection of preclinical cancer *in apparently well women*, when the disease is unsuspected by patient or physician, as is possible in mass screening for the disease.

3. Breast cancer is an insidious disease that may be present and may develop over many years without signs or symptoms of any kind. Every woman over thirty or thirty-five years of age who visits a physician for any medical condition or only for a checkup must be regarded as possibly harboring a breast cancer.

In other words, the success of breast-cancer treatment may depend on the stage at which intervention is introduced. If breast cancer is found and treated when localized, and before the immune system has been compromised, the cure rate may be high. The optimum time for detection at the most curable stage may be before the woman is aware of a problem or even before the lesion is palpable by woman or physician. Such cancers may be detectable only through the mass screening of women from the age of thirty-five onward.

HOW SHOULD WE DO MASS SCREENING?

The basic procedures used in mass screening are:

1. An interview to develop demographic data, such as ethnic background, education, parity (childbearing),

and menstrual and breast history, in order to develop clues to increased risk.

2. A careful clinical examination by a physician well versed in the procedure or by a properly trained paramedical person under the guidance of a clinician.

3. Teaching of breast self-examination (BSE), preferably on a one-to-one basis, and convincing the woman of the need to do it regularly. Because none of the methods for detection of a breast cancer is 100 percent accurate, women have to be made aware that a cancer may become detectable within a few months after a presumably negative examination; we call this an *interval* cancer. Reliance must be placed on breast self-examination to fill the time gap. Every woman should, therefore, be made familiar with the procedure for BSE, preferably at the time of clinical examination. (Mass screening offers an excellent opportunity for such education of women.) BSE makes possible detection of the interval cancer at an earlier, more curable stage.

4. Mammography, or soft-tissue X-ray examination of the breast. This procedure, which is at least seventy years old, has been considerably refined and brought to a high degree of technical excellence. Use of special machines and fast films produces mammograms of excellent quality with markedly reduced radiation dosage—down from 8 to 12 rads to less than 0.5 rad to the skin and less than 0.05 rad to the midbreast for the two views generally used, a very minute dose indeed! Many radiologists use their regular X-ray equipment with a Xerox process, producing images on charged selenium-coated aluminum plates and ending with mammograms on special paper. This method also produces breast im-

ages of excellent quality, although with radiation dosage to the breast about six to eight times that of modern film-screen combinations. There are strong advocates of both methods. Both methods can produce images of the proper quality, as long as the radiologist develops the necessary expertise and dedication to the procedure. Adequate visualization of the breast, with fine detail and contrast, is vital for accuracy. A less than fully adequate film may lead to a false diagnosis.

It is important to mention that a breast cancer may still be in the very early stages and not be palpable by even the most expert hands. The occult cancer, completely *asymptomatic* and *nonpalpable*, is detectable only by mammography.

It should also be emphasized that because neither palpation nor mammography is 100 percent accurate, if cancer is suspected on palpation, a negative mammogram should never be allowed to delay exploration of a breast. Similarly, a clinician who is faced with negative clinical findings, but with a positive mammographic report, should seriously consider exploration. The two modalities are complementary. They should never be considered competitive.

The improved mammographic techniques have resulted in a substantial increase in cancers found on mammography. Improvement in technique has continued and is continuing. And yet less than 15 percent of women in this country have ever had a mammogram or the type of proper palpation needed to detect changes. What are the problems, and how can we solve them? How can women be helped to take advantage of the opportunities for screening?

HOSPITAL CENTER VS. COMMUNITY CENTER

There is a difference of opinion about where a fixed screening facility should be located. Many presumably well women prefer a screening center set up under community auspices and located in the community, but not in association with a hospital. Financial considerations in some areas would suggest that a community center could be operated with less financial overhead than a hospital-based center. This type of question has to be resolved on a local level. It should also be borne in mind that many women may prefer to have the complete periodic breast examination performed under the auspices of their private physician. Individual needs in this regard must be considered, especially when cost of examination is concerned.

MOBILE VAN VS. FIXED CENTER

Over the years, mobile vans with the proper equipment aboard have been used to bring the procedure to women, particularly in low-income areas or in regions far removed from a fixed facility. Such vans have been successful in introducing screening examinations to women who needed them but would otherwise not be in a position to have them. It is important to realize that such mobile screening should maintain an "umbilical cord" to a fixed center to allow further investigation of problem cases and to arrange for periodic checkups. Many women will take advantage of a mobile checkup in their own neighborhood, especially if the fixed center is in a hospital which they may be afraid to approach on their own. However, the fixed center, with its facilities for physical examination, would appear to be a most important backup.

SYMPTOMATIC VS. ASYMPTOMATIC

Theoretically, mass screening for breast cancer should involve the presumably well woman who has no abnormal breast signs or symptoms. Therein, however, lies our dilemma. The usual breast symptoms—a lump or lumps, diffused or localized pain, nipple discharge —that would classify a woman as "symptomatic" are present to some degree in all women. The distinction between "symptomatic" and "asymptomatic" is quite blurred. Does a woman with the usual lumpiness, with perhaps one or more lumps that stand out, qualify as "symptomatic"? Is the woman with premenstrual swelling or pain of varying degree "asymptomatic"? In truth, every woman has breast symptoms or signs of varying severity. Since breast cancer is often present without signs or symptoms, is it not more useful to consider all women as "symptomatic" and to offer screening to all women—except perhaps those already under the care of a physician for a particular problem?

WHAT AGE TO START?

Some question the benefit of screening women who are under fifty years of age. Preliminary data from the HIP study led statisticians to question the mortality benefit in that study in women under the age of fifty. However, up-to-date statistics from eighteen years of follow-up indicate a reduction in mortality of about 25 percent in women under fifty as well as in those over fifty. These most recent data should dispel notions that screening should be done only in women over fifty. It is hoped that the benefits of early detection can thus be extended to all women who are at risk for getting the disease. Certainly all women over forty should be given the opportunity not only to get the reassurance that they are well, but also the potential of curability if a cancer is indeed present.

To sum up the case for mass screening of women:

1. Most women with breast cancer could be saved by detection of the disease in an early, more curable stage if physicians would teach their patients to examine their breasts properly once a month and—this is most important—encourage them to have complete, periodic breast examinations to include mammography.

2. It is now time to allay concerns about the risk involved in screening procedures. More attention should now be paid to the remaining problems in screening: The costs of screening; detection of true high-risk factors; and methods for improving women's motivation to seek screening. The problem of breast cancer as the number one cancer in women is still very much with us. We know from present evidence that detection of early breast cancer results not only in increased survival, but in the possibility of much smaller surgical procedures. It is therefore imperative that we move ahead with screening activities by making them more effective, more practical, and more acceptable to all women and their physicians.

8

HOW BREAST CANCER IS TREATED

In recent years there has been much controversy in the media—newspapers and magazines, radio and television—about how much or how little surgery is desirable in breast cancer. Discussion has been generated by different schools of thought, all with influential adherents and all with weighty arguments. Unfortunately, the data presented by each side are not acceptable to the other, so that differences of opinion remain. The woman with possible breast cancer finds herself in the middle without knowing which way to turn.

Mrs. B.S., aged thirty-six, mother of three, nudged her husband at 3:00 A.M. "Jack, I think I feel a lump in

my right breast!" She was terrified. The next morning
her suspicions were confirmed by her physician. A surgical colleague verified the need for a biopsy, the removal of the growth for accurate diagnosis.

"We just have to explore to find out," he said.

"Could it be a cancer?" she asked tremulously.

"Yes, it may well be," he answered.

"What will you do then?" she asked quietly.

"We shall then have to remove your breast."

"Will you talk the matter over with me before you
take that step?"

"No, the biopsy specimen will be examined by the
pathologist by what we call a frozen section, while you
are asleep. If diagnosis of cancer is made, we shall proceed with a mastectomy—a removal of the breast."

"Can't I have a chance to wake up and think it over?"

"No, I would prefer to have your consent to proceed
in advance. It is not best for you, in my judgment, to
delay and return to the operating room for a second
operation. I believe it is better to do the necessary surgery as soon as a diagnosis is established."

"I've been reading about doctors who are inclined to
do less surgery and even try to save most of the breast.
They insist that a woman should have the right to decide
in an important matter like this what she wants to have
done to her body. I'd like to have that chance even if
another operation is necessary later."

"I agree that you have the right to decide—that is
why we are discussing the matter. But if you insist on
two operations, I must advise you to seek another surgeon. I cannot in good conscience do what you wish."

Mrs. B.S. had heard of a surgeon who would agree
with her ideas. She did seek his opinion. She did have
less than a mastectomy for her breast cancer. However,

the intense emotional upheaval, the anxieties and fears connected with her illness, the possibility that she had made a wrong decision, the thought that she may therefore be doomed—all these have weighed heavily on her and her family. Many other women, on the other hand, go along with the decision to do the usual extensive surgery and then go through the agony of wondering whether less disfiguring surgery would have been adequate.

It has been calculated that there are perhaps fourteen treatment combinations possible for a woman with breast cancer. Opinions differ widely among the experts in this country as well as abroad. Treatments vary all the way from a needle diagnosis followed by radiation therapy to supraradical surgery—and many combinations in between. Prominent surgeons have gone on record as sincerely and strongly favoring one form of treatment over another. When we add such procedures as oophorectomy (removal of the ovaries), chemotherapy (chemical treatments during or after operation), and radiation therapy before or after surgery, the possible combinations are literally legion. Clinical trials are being done here and abroad to evaluate several treatment methods to find the best answer. Dr. Bernard Fisher of Pittsburgh is in charge of one complex study to evaluate different combinations of treatment. Early conclusions from his ongoing studies strongly suggest that less than removal of the entire breast does just as well as complete mastectomy, particularly if the cancer is detected in an early stage. It may take many years to reach generally acceptable conclusions.

The probability remains that honest differences of opinion will continue to exist because patients are in different stages of the disease when they come to phy-

sicians, and because physicians are, after all, only human beings with special expertise but with highly individual psychological backgrounds and skills.

In the welter of confusion stimulated by articles urging that women have a right to make a decision about the extent of surgery to be performed on their bodies, no one seems to realize that the woman involved has no real scientific basis for making a judgment. How can a woman plagued by intense anxiety and lack of knowledge decide what type of surgical procedure should be undertaken for her own breast cancer? The truth of the matter is that we are begging the question. Every woman with breast cancer must make the only decision she is capable of making: She must choose which physician will be responsible for her treatment; she cannot choose which treatment to have. She must rely completely on the good judgment of the physician in whom she has confidence.

The medical profession will eventually have to come to grips with the general problem of more or less surgery, and, more important, specifically for the particular woman—with all her personal problems and needs— who is entrusting her fate to her physician's hands. The humane and expert surgeon considers his patient as a whole human being and not as just a breast cancer. He adjusts his procedure not only to the type of cancer present but also to the emotional and mental makeup of his patient. The procedure must be suited to the individual.

In this controversy, however, the most significant fact is often overlooked—and that is the stage of the disease when it is detected and treated. All clinicians interested in treatment of breast cancer are agreed that the most important ingredient is what is called "an early lesion."

All surgeons hope that every cancer of the breast coming in for treatment will be an early one—one that is localized to the breast, one that is so small it is felt hardly or not at all by their expert fingers. That is the cancer they can cure, and the one that may lead, we hope, to less surgery. When we reach the time when most breast cancer is found in the curable stage, controversy over the extent of surgery will lessen. For the more or less late cancers that are now found all too often, surgeons feel they must use mastectomy to give the woman the best chance for a cure. When these same sincere surgeons are faced with more of the small, curable variety, they will be glad to do less surgery and end up with a woman who remains emotionally healthy as well as cured of her cancer.

Physicians responsible for the care of breast cancer are acutely aware of the following:

- Surgical treatment offers the best hope for a cure. It may be combined with other forms of treatment, but removal of all the cancer remains the basis for best results.
- Too many women still visit their physicians for the first time with far advanced breast cancer—too far advanced for successful treatment. A few years ago it was estimated that one-third of breast cancers in the United States were so far advanced that they were considered inoperable—too late for surgery.
- Surgical treatment is effective when the cancer is still confined to the breast. When the armpit glands are involved, cures are fewer. Long-term survival is related to the amount of involvement beyond the breast.
- Many surgeons in this country and elsewhere still feel strongly that a complete removal of the breast and

adjacent potentially involved structures—radical mastectomy—is the best treatment for operable breast cancer. A growing vociferous minority is opting for less extensive surgery in the presence of small cancers—some are even advocating less than total removal of the breast. Studies have been under way for several years in the United States, England, Canada and Italy that are shedding light on this problem. Many surgeons are doing much less extensive procedures as a result.

Cancer is an insidious disease. It starts on a microscopic level and then infiltrates and invades normal adjacent structures to become a mass which then discards the local controls. It then sends out scouts to set up colonies in other vital organs to continue its growth. The regional glands (lymph nodes) act as a defense mechanism, or barrier, to prevent the metastasis from spreading elsewhere. Unfortunately, the filtering mechanism itself tends to become cancerous. For this reason the glands in the armpit or under the breastbone may be removed.

The aim of the surgical procedure is the removal of all tissue invaded by cancer. For the past seventy-five years the dictum in the surgical management of cancer of the breast has been "Remove all the breast involved with cancer and the regional lymph glands filtering the cancer." Because the chest muscles (or pectoralis major and minor) extend across the armpit, and because their covering may also be involved with the adjacent nodes, they are removed together with the breast and the armpit glands. This operation is known as a *radical mastectomy*. When the cancer is in the inner half of the breast

and there is a likelihood that the glands under the breastbone are involved, a few surgeons will remove these glands, too—the *supraradical mastectomy*.

Many surgeons, now perhaps in the majority, have been leaving the chest muscles so that there is less chest deformity after the operation. This procedure is called *modified radical mastectomy*. Under certain conditions, such as weakened general physical condition or in very early cases, a surgeon may remove only the breast proper, leaving muscles and glands intact. This procedure is known as a *simple mastectomy* or *total mastectomy*.

Over the years a few daring surgeons in some countries have felt that removal of less than the entire breast would suffice, especially in the early and small cancers with which there is no apparent involvement of the armpit. This operation, known variously as *wide local excision, partial mastectomy, lumpectomy,* or *tylectomy,* is usually followed by radiation therapy to the remaining breast tissue and neighboring lymph glands. The advocates of mastectomy point out that thorough microscopic studies have shown that in as many as 90 percent of obvious cancers there are other seeds of cancer elsewhere in the breast which are not detectable by ordinary examination, and that partial removal of a breast may leave cancer behind. Those with an opposite view point out that radiation therapy is probably effective for these early seeds of cancer, if present, and that with modern methods of detection one might safely observe the breast and postpone more surgery till the disease again becomes apparent. It should be emphasized that before extensive surgery is undertaken, a biopsy is made. A small piece of tissue is removed for microscopic study and a definite diagnosis. Sometimes the specimen is

X-rayed to make sure that the proper area has been removed and is being studied. This procedure is called *specimen radiography*.

Another form of treatment for breast cancer is *radiation therapy*, using various forms of sophisticated equipment. This is usually reserved for postsurgical situations in which cancer is suspected as still being present. It may be used to treat glands that might be involved but which have not been removed. It is known that breast cancer, especially in early stages, is sensitive to the X ray. However, some cancers do not respond as well as others. It is difficult, if not impossible, to know which types will be completely destroyed. X-ray therapy is also used to treat areas of metastasis or spread. It is often used as the sole treatment in advanced forms of the disease that are not operable.

Hormone therapy is based on the fact that breast cancer is in some way associated with the secretions from endocrine glands, especially the "sex hormones." Manipulation of the sex-hormone environment of the body— by surgical removal of the ovaries, the adrenals, and the pituitary, or by giving special hormones or anti-hormones to the patient—often produces remarkable long-term control.

Chemotherapy is treatment with cancer-killing drugs. Many drugs have been tried, some with great success, in breast cancer. New ones are regularly being produced. These drugs can indeed destroy much of the cancer, but usually not its entirety. There is still a great need for the "magic bullet" that will destroy all cancer cells wherever they may be hiding but will not be harmful to normal cells.

An important part of the story of breast-cancer treatment is rehabilitation. Because the mainstay of current treatment is surgical and often involves extensive procedures, physical and emotional problems are common. Great strides have been made in overcoming them. The American Cancer Society has been in the forefront of such activities. Its "Reach to Recovery" program, originated and stimulated by a tireless, farsighted, and compassionate woman, Therese Lasser, has brought to many women the comfort and reassurance that a normal life—emotionally as well as physically—can today follow breast surgery.

The program is conducted on a national basis by a group of dedicated volunteers who themselves have had mastectomies, and who are trained in the proper approach to a woman who has had recent surgery. After receiving the approval of the attending surgeon, they usually visit the patient before she has left the hospital; help her to develop an optimistic outlook on her condition; give her the reassurance that her life can remain sexually, socially, and emotionally as before; and leave information on proper exercises. They also provide a temporary prosthesis so that the woman can leave the hospital in the same outfit she wore when she came in.

In most cases, proper well-fitting bras and prostheses, as well as carefully regulated exercises, can bring to postsurgical women normal appearance, normal activity, and normal social relationships.

9

WHAT ELSE PHYSICIANS COULD DO

Many questions have been raised. New roads have been charted for future progress in the continuing fight against breast cancer. Much remains to be done by physicians and much remains to be done by you. Let us consider first what more could be done by the medical profession.

Our greatest efforts must be directed to learning more about what causes breast cancer. Are there factors that can be controlled? One school of thought believes that two different sets of factors may be operating—one that starts the process and another that promotes its growth. Some think that diet (particularly fats) has an effect in promoting cancer growth. A project has been started in the Netherlands to see if weight reduction may have a beneficial effect in reducing the risk of developing breast cancer.

Is there a virus involved—a submicroscopic living substance that changes the programming in a cell and turns it into an enemy of its neighbors? If so—and there is evidence that this occurs in some animals, such as mice—can this substance be isolated and a vaccine produced against it? Someday, perhaps, girl babies may be immunized against breast cancer. Such a concept would take much time and effort to substantiate. Even if a successful vaccine were produced, a whole generation of women would still be at risk and would still require all our efforts at earlier detection and treatment. Until the time when we learn to prevent the disease from developing at all, we must continue to try to prevent disability and death.

When we have found the remedy that will eradicate the disease regardless of the stage in which it is detected, the pressure for earlier detection will be lessened. The probability is that such a remedy will lie in a still unknown chemical or a still unknown ability to manipulate the hormonal or immunological defense mechanism of the body. In the meantime we must use our surgical, radiotherapeutic, and chemotherapeutic tools to the best of our ability. Today this means finding breast cancer when it is confined to the breast or has only minimal spread. The earlier in its development the cancer is detected and the smaller its size, the greater our success with our present remedies. With our improved devices, we can find breast cancer when we can cure the woman, which is more than can be said of many other forms of cancer. We must continue to take advantage of this fact.

In the meantime we must continue to develop methods of diagnosis that are more accurate, more economical, and less time-consuming. We must find ways of tracking down the enemy when it is even smaller than we now find it. We must develop ever finer sieves so that it will not slip by as it now does too often.

Of great interest, too, would be improved methods of identifying high-risk populations. We have made only little progress in this direction. If we could find those women who are substantially more likely to develop breast cancer, we could concentrate on them and examine them more frequently. At the same time, we could conserve our time and energy and examine the low-risk women less frequently.

For many years, oncologists (cancer specialists) have believed that hormones, particularly estrogens, produced by the ovaries or adrenal glands were in some way closely associated with breast cancer. It has been known for some time that estrogens in substantial amounts could produce breast cancer in susceptible mice. The relationship to breast cancer in humans, however, has been much less clear. For instance, it is known that during many months of pregnancy the amounts of estrogen in the body increase to very high levels—up to ten times the usual amount—yet breast cancer seldom develops during pregnancy. Estrogen has been used for years to treat change-of-life symptoms such as flushes, dizziness, and depression. Tons of these hormones have been taken by thousands of women for long periods of time. Yet the incidence of breast cancer has not increased remarkably.

Much investigation is going on in this area of female hormone production and its involvement in breast conditions. The whole field is exciting and may offer biochemical clues to a better understanding of the cause of breast cancer.

An intriguing area for determining high-risk factors is evaluation of the emotional life of a woman. It is well known that psychological factors have a powerful effect on the endocrine system. Could such factors play a part in the hormone development of the young female and make her more or less likely to develop a subsequent breast cancer? Could a psychological questionnaire be constructed that would detect such factors? There are experts in the breast field who think such a possibility exists and should be investigated.

A most important problem that needs to be studied is motivation. How does one stimulate women to accept, if not demand the *complete* breast examination? Motivation is more easily developed in higher-income groups. But how about the minority groups or those at lower-income levels? How can they be made aware of the breast-cancer problem and how can they be brought in for examination? Such an effort requires education and dissemination of information at the community level, perhaps even on a personal level. Perhaps it will be necessary to keep screening centers open at night or on weekends to accommodate working mothers. Subcenters may need to be established in the communities where low-income women live. Other communities should follow the lead of the Guttman Institute, which operated a 26-foot mobile unit that contained all the advanced equipment necessary for a complete examination, and moved from one neighborhood to another. Special mobile equipment for mammography is also available that can be transported to locations for health fairs and community screening sessions. More emphasis must be placed on the use of trained paramedical personnel to examine large numbers of women.

In short, until we learn how to protect ourselves against the onset and development of breast cancer, we must continue to use improved methods of detection and treatment to cure the disease more often. We must also tell more women that much of their protection lies in their own hands. And the American Cancer Society must be supported in its continuing programs of education and information.

10

ALL WOMEN NEED THESE EXAMINATIONS— WHY HAVEN'T THEY HAD THEM?

Our improved techniques of breast examination for detection of breast cancer have resulted in more cancers found in a curable stage than ever before. The examinations are safe, accurate, and painless. Yet most women of the proper age have not had even one mammogram. What are the psychological and practical barriers and how can we overcome them? Here is a list of the major obstacles that still prevent early detection:

FEAR OF RESULT

The fear of finding a cancer is a stumbling block faced by many women. The anxiety connected with an examination frightens many women away from a possibly lifesaving procedure. Women need to be assured and reassured that the main goal of screening is to make sure they do *not* have breast cancer. Subsequent periodic examinations can help them remain free of the disease. They must be constantly assured and reassured that the vast majority of women—at least nine out of ten—will end up with the pleasant knowledge that all is well. They must be assured and reassured that if a woman does have a problem, it will be detected in an early curable stage so that the treatment will not only save her life but very often her breast as well.

FEAR OF X RAYS

For many years, it has been known that the breast is sensitive to X rays. In 1976, statements were made and reported at length in the media that mammography, which uses X rays, might in itself produce breast cancer, and that the hazard might be greater than the benefit. Concern over hazard from X-radiation in mammography has been sadly overrated and has led to unnecessary and unreasonable fear that the procedure itself could cause harm. Many women all over the country at that time refused to have mammograms, and many cancers went undetected in the more curable stage. Unfortunately, many women will still die because of this refusal.

Many studies by authorities have concluded that the risk from mammography, if any, is dependent on the age of the woman and the dose of X rays given. There is no evidence of significant hazard in women over thirty-five—the age at which periodic mass screening is suggested. The dose from modern mammography continues to be reduced and is so small—down to less than 0.05 rad to the midbreast—that any hazard from periodic mammography, even over many years, must be considered negligible and probably not even measurable. Certainly the potential benefit from mammography far exceeds any remote hazard.

COST OF EXAMINATION

Cost of examination, including mammography, is of little importance when examining the comparatively few women who truly show a possible problem. However, when large numbers of asymptomatic or minimally symptomatic women are involved, as in mass screening, especially when they are in a low income bracket, the cost of the procedures, particularly that of mammography, becomes important. In general, community mass screening should involve, if possible, the use of dedicated personnel under the auspices of a nonprofit or low-profit center, using many volunteers and medical personnel imbued with a sense of dedication and even personal sacrifice for the satisfaction of saving women's lives. A few such centers are in operation in this country and act as examples of what can be done when the will and proper attitude are available. Noteworthy are the Guttman Institute in New York City, where a minimal charge of $45.00 is made, and the Strax Institute in Lauderhill, Florida, where a similar charge is made for the complete examination, including thorough clinical examination as well as mammography.

It should be emphasized that low-cost mass screening requires the involvement of large numbers of women— at least 10,000 per year. It also requires the dedication of community leaders as well as that of physicians in the area, the cooperation of women's groups, and possibly the operation of the screening activities under community auspices rather than those of a "for-profit" institution. Soliciting the cooperation of third-party payers is also important.

OTHER WAYS OF TESTING

Because mammography uses ionizing radiation, which has produced concern in some quarters that it may be carcinogenic to the breast, other procedures have been introduced, presumably to replace mammography. However, it has been found by various radiologists, and emphasized by the American College of Radiology, that only mammography is capable of detecting the nonpalpable cancer. Procedures like thermography, sonography, diaphanography, magnetic-resonance, or aspiration biopsy, can be useful in providing additional information on a palpable mass. But since one of our important activities in mass screening is detection of breast cancer in a nonpalpable stage, experts suggest that mammography is the only reliable method of breast imaging for use in mass screening.

MOTIVATION

Perhaps the most important factor in making mass screening successful is motivation of women to accept the procedure. Success in saving lives through mass screening is in direct proportion to the numbers of women who participate. We must use the hysteria about breast cancer, as evidenced by the media and exaggerated in the minds of women, to stimulate women to accept and even demand mass screening. They must insist on such procedures through public health authorities as well as through their own physicians. If mass screening is the only means we have to save lives from the disease, women's groups must be in the forefront to demand such procedures as their right. Physicians must be made to realize that it is their duty to alert women to the danger and to make possible the tests that are necessary to overcome the disease.

Efforts in this direction must be ongoing and persistent and relate to the population involved. The educational feature of mass screening varies in different communities among women of different ethnic groups and cultural backgrounds. Awareness of progress needs to be promoted. The centers for such screening must be

readily available and easily accessible. The American
Cancer Society and its volunteers have had an excellent
input into such activities by making available use of the
media and by stimulating direct neighborhood efforts.
Women's organizations, such as the U.O.T.S., which
are particularly interested in this type of activity, can be
most helpful.

When women learn through screening that no disease
is present, they receive a tremendous psychological benefit. The likelihood that they *will* be reassured should
be a strong factor motivating them to participate in widespread mass screening.

RISK FACTORS

Mass screening to detect possible breast cancers in asymptomatic or minimally symptomatic women is a difficult
goal. A thousand women need to be examined to find
perhaps a half-dozen cancers. The current prevalence
rate—depending on the age of the women, parity (childbearing), and even preselection by the screenees—*may
be less than 1 percent*. Today, three out of four cancers
are detected in women who have none of the usually
mentioned risk factors, according to American Cancer
Society statisticians. The two factors indicating highest
risk—a personal history of cancer in one breast or a
positive family history involving a premenopausal
mother or sister, especially with bilateral breast cancer
—are found in a very small percentage of women. Yet
we must consider all women over thirty-five to be at
risk for having or getting breast cancer.

DEGREE OF COMPRESSION IN MAMMOGRAPHY

It is well known that optimal technique in mammography is vital for best results. How can one get the best results? Compression of the breast has been used for many years as a means of producing better detail with less chance of missing important abnormalities. This is particularly true in the postmenopausal or large breast.

However, a problem has recently surfaced. Modern mammography devices include a compression plate, which cannot always be controlled or regulated by the technician. Many breasts are quite sensitive, and the insistence by the technician or radiologist on vigorous compression of the breast has produced vociferous complaints and even many bruised breasts. Careful study of the program indicates that vigorous compression is usually not at all necessary for proper detail and visualization, and that this type of compression will turn women away from a potentially lifesaving procedure. The attending radiologist, and particularly the technician, must learn to treat each woman as an individual and apply compression as judiciously as possible in each particular case. The average-sized breast certainly does not require vigorous compression for proper delineation of breast structure.

All these considerations have led to new guidelines for the use of mammography; the guidelines have been issued by the American Cancer Society with the concurrence of the American College of Radiology and the American Academy of Family Physicians. They are as follows:

1. All women with signs and symptoms of breast disease should have a mammogram as well as a physician's examination as often and whenever needed, regardless of age.
2. All women should have a base-line mammogram between the ages of thirty-five and forty, whether symptomatic or not.
3. All women between forty and fifty should have a physical examination annually, and mammography every year, or at least every two years.
4. All women over fifty should have both a physical examination and mammography every year.

11

WHAT ELSE YOU CAN DO? TEN PRECEPTS FOR PROTECTION

A set of precepts for the modern woman who would like to do all she can to protect herself from breast cancer, for her own sake and for those dear to her, should include the following:

- Remember that breast cancer is a curable disease—if caught in time.

- Note that we have the methods and equipment to detect breast cancer in its early stages when it is still confined to the breast and is therefore curable.
- Be aware of the enemy and realize that you have powerful methods on your side.
- Your most valuable weapon is your own hands. Use them properly and regularly once a month in doing breast self-examination.
- Visit your physician once a year—or more frequently if he or she finds it advisable—for a complete examination. Such an examination may require more equipment and expertise than the physician has. If so, ask for special studies to be arranged.
- Remember that most breast conditions are harmless. At the same time, remember that you owe it to yourself to inform your physician of any new findings in your breast, for only he or she can make the proper differential diagnosis.
- Alert all women close to you to the above advice, and urge them to follow through.
- Learn as much as you can about the breast and its disorders. Ask questions of your physician if you do not understand. The more knowledge you have, the better you can protect yourself. Keep informed about new discoveries—you never know when they may be useful.
- Never take lightly a change in your breasts. The reassurance of a negative examination (one that does not show the presence of cancer) is worth more than the effort involved in getting it.
- Above all, remember that the odds are strongly against your ever developing breast cancer—*but* that you must be on your guard at all times.

12

ON THE
HORIZON

Our ultimate goal in the battle against cancer is primary prevention of the basic cancer process. Much effort has been expended by microbiologists and cancer investigators all over the world in this direction. Unfortunately, no major breakthrough can be predicted for the near future.

A more directed approach involves the general concept that cancer of an organ is in a practical sense unique to that organ, not to the body as a whole. This leads to the idea that the basic cancer change in the cell—the oncogene—may well be an inherited process and may be fundamentally the same for all cancer, but that its effect and proliferation are unique for the organ it involves. Therefore, the development of the oncogene in any particular organ may depend on different promoting factors that can lead to the particular cancer in that organ and may well be different for cancers of different organs. This thought in turn leads to the idea that if we could identify more clearly the promoting factors, two practical benefits might result:

1. We could isolate some basic promoting factors which, if easily identified, could lead to a particular screening process. This, in turn, could lead to identifying a group of people at high risk for the cancer in question. Screening efforts could then be emphasized for those truly at risk.
2. If there is evidence that early detection of a cancer would lower mortality, we would indeed have a more practical method for early detection and for saving of lives from the particular cancer. Even more, such a situation could lead to removal of the important promoting factors and thus to secondary prevention by preventing the development of the disease.

When we consider the major types of cancer—such as that of the breast, lung, cervix or colon—this type of reasoning leads to a few important clues to the problem:

WHAT TRIGGERS THE ONCOGENES?

We know of some risk factors that lead to increased prevalence of a particular cancer. For example, we know that nulliparity (childlessness in a woman), early menarche, or late menopause are important risk factors for breast cancer. We know that smoking and exposure to asbestos or other pollutants are risk factors for lung cancer. We know that promiscuity or early sexual activity, particularly with uncircumcised males, presents added risk for cervical cancer. We know a low-fiber diet and constipation pose added risk for colon cancer. We also know that in all of these situations, a positive family history—where cancer has occurred in family members —looms large in our evaluation of risk.

However, in breast cancer, over 75 percent of women who develop the disease have none of the above risk factors. Also, most women who have the risk factors do not develop the disease. It is also true that most heavy smokers do not develop lung cancer and that lung cancer does indeed develop in people who are not exposed to the risk factors mentioned. The same reasoning holds for the other cancers listed above. Most people who are on a low-fiber diet do not develop colon cancer, and most women who are sexually promiscuous do not develop cervical cancer.

All this would suggest that cancer may be a two-step process. The initial cause may be an abnormal gene that is programmed to bring on the cancer. The development of a particular cancer, as we know it, may well be an inherited factor that relates to a specific organ—be it breast or cervix or lung or colon. If this gene is present but none of the so-called risk factors or secondary causes are present, no cancer may develop. Conversely, if risk factors are present but no oncogene is about, no cancer will develop. The combination of both is essential to the development of the disease. Perhaps, too, the degrees of abnormality or multiplicity of the oncogenes may play a part in early development. Also, a weak oncogene combined with multiple exaggerated risk factors may lead to the disease.

Much effort has been expended in typing the oncogenes for the common cancers. An actual benefit from such endeavors still eludes us. If on the other hand, we could authoritatively delineate the risk factors, we would be ahead. This could lead us to a screening program for early detection—if such early detection has been proved to actually reduce mortality, as is the case in breast cancer. However, not only do we need to know the risk factors, but we need to speculate or know how such risk factors could produce the irritation or the spark that would stimulate the oncogene to its nefarious activity. For example, if in breast cancer we could delineate the true risk factor which is a result of a change on a fundamental level, such as endocrine abnormality or change in metabolism, we could then use that true risk factor to help us concentrate our screening activities on a limited group and make screening efforts more practical than at present. But, even more important, such success might make it possible to remove or delete or change the risk factor and prevent the development of the disease.

HORMONAL FACTORS

It is almost obvious that the hormone makeup of a woman must relate strongly to the promotion of breast cancer and that dietary factors may be important through their effect on the hormones. Many investigators have found bits of evidence that such a relationship may indeed be the case. The leads seem to have narrowed down to estrogen and its fractions, progesterone and prolactin, as being singly or in combination deeply involved in the process.

Since excellent and accurate methods have been developed for determination of these hormones, it seemed reasonable to conduct a large-scale prospective study to evaluate these substances and relate them to the detection of breast cancer. Such a study has been under way under the auspices of the department of Environmental Medicine of the New York University Medical Center and the Guttman and Strax institutes, in cooperation with investigators from the Imperial Cancer Research Fund of Great Britain and the Netherlands Cancer Institute. The project may have two important potentials: It may tell us whether there is a truly high-risk group of women, and if the increased risk is related to an abnormal ratio of the hormones, as is strongly hinted at by several investigators. With such results, the potential of primary prevention by correcting the abnormality becomes exciting. To this end, a study has been funded by the National Cancer Institute to investigate "Endocrine and Environmental Factors in Breast Cancer."

It is thought that in three to four years, perhaps by 1992 or 1993, we will have the information we are looking for—that is, *we will know from the blood hormone picture which woman is really at risk for getting a breast cancer.* We will then be able to make our screening efforts much more practical, and we may have developed the possibility of preventing breast cancer.

PSYCHOSOCIAL FACTORS

Another study has been mounted to investigate "Psychosocial Factors" involved in the development of breast cancer. These factors—especially stress; personality traits or coping styles; and personal habits and risk behaviors—may be very important to the development of the disease through their effect on the hormones. Since we are already collecting hormonal information on the women in the blood study, it should not be difficult to obtain information on psychosocial factors by asking them to fill out a questionnaire at the same time we take the blood. Should the role of psychological factors be further clarified, then these factors could offer us an important opportunity to intervene for cancer control in areas that are amenable to easily administered behavioral techniques.

13

DO YOU HAVE A QUESTION?

Q. *How many women get breast cancer each year?*

A. The National Cancer Institute estimates that in 1989 about 142,000 American women will be diagnosed with breast cancer and 43,022 will die of the disease. One out of ten women will develop the disease in her lifetime.

Q. *How many breast-cancer patients are premenopausal?*

A. About 25 percent (35,000 estimated in 1989) of all breast cancers are in women under age fifty.

Q. *How do I know if I'm at higher risk for getting breast cancer?*

A. You are at a higher risk for getting breast cancer if you are in any of the following categories: you have already had one breast cancer; you have a mother or sister who had breast cancer before her change of life; you have had no children; you are in an upper economic bracket. However, and it should be emphasized, the vast majority of women who have any of these risk factors will *not* get breast cancer. Also, three out of four women who do get breast cancer have none of these risk factors.

Q. *What can I do to prevent getting breast cancer?*

A. We do not know. There is some evidence that women after the menopause should have *low-fat* diets. Methods for prevention still elude us. Perhaps the studies referred to in Chapter 11, "On the Horizon," will shed some light on the subject.

Q. *Where can I get a mammogram?*

A. Ask your doctor or, if need be, ask your local American Cancer Society chapter.

Q. *I have a lump in my breast. What should I do?*

A. See your doctor as soon as possible. If he suggests further examinations, by all means, follow through.

Q. *Is breast cancer contagious?*

A. Not at all. There is no evidence whatsoever that such is the case.

Q. *Does radiation cause breast cancer?*

A. There is some evidence that very large doses of X-radiation can stimulate the growth of breast cancer. However, the radiation that is used in breast examination by modern mammography is so minute that all authorities feel that if there is any risk at all, it must be negligible and cannot even be measured.

Q. *Do implant procedures pose a risk for developing breast cancer?*

A. There is absolutely no evidence that modern techniques with implants lead to increased breast-cancer risk. Injection of silicone does, however, cause problems, but this is virtually not done anymore. All women should have regular breast examinations, especially if they have had any surgical procedures on their breasts.

Q. *My mother had breast cancer. Does that mean that I'll probably get it too?*

A. Only one in ten American women develops breast cancer. If your mother, sister, or maternal aunt has had breast cancer and if she developed the disease before her change of life, your chance of developing the disease is about twice that of a woman without such a history. If, however, the cancer developed after the menopause, your risk is only slightly elevated. You must, however, be certain to examine your breasts regularly and see your physician periodically for a thorough breast examination. Should you or your physician find any change in your breast, more frequent examination and other diagnostic procedures may be indicated.

Q. *I was struck violently on the breast. It became discolored and a lump developed which gradually disappeared. Could such an injury lead to breast cancer?*

A. No, there is absolutely no evidence that injury or manipulation as may occur in lovemaking has any connection with breast cancer. The breast, because of its exposed position, is subject to many bumps and bruises which heal completely, although a lump may persist for an indeterminate time and gradually disappear. All lumps, however, should be checked by your physician promptly.

Q. *I have had breast cancer. I have a grown daughter. What precautions should she take, if any?*

A. Although her risk of developing a breast cancer may be increased, she should face the situation without fear. After all, the odds remain very much against her developing the disease. After her breasts begin to develop, she should learn to examine her breasts and be checked by her physician regularly. After thirty-five, mammography should be added. She should inform her physician promptly of any change that she may find at any time between examinations.

Q. *I have heard that nursing a baby protects one against breast cancer. Is that true?*

A. It used to be thought that breast-feeding—especially prolonged breast-feeding—was associated with a lower incidence of breast cancer. The latest data on a worldwide basis refute this concept. Apparently there is no relationship between nursing and breast cancer.

Q. *All my life I have had very large breasts. After my meno-pause, they became larger. Do I run a greater risk of getting a cancer?*

A. Size of breast has no relation to breast cancer. The large-breasted woman should be watched more closely with a complete examination, because a small mass may be undetected for a longer time in a very large breast. Mammography is a good diagnostic method for the large breast, which usually contains much fat in which small masses are more readily visible than in a breast with less fat.

Q. *I have had a watery discharge from my right nipple for the past few months. I have no pain or other discomfort. Is it cause for concern?*

A. Slight nipple discharges are not unusual. They are due to duct irritations and have no connection with the development of breast cancer. They may be thin or thick, colorless, white, yellow, or green. Such breasts should, of course, be evaluated by a physician. Discharges are ordinarily no cause for concern unless they are conspicuously bloody or clear yellow. However, physicians will check the breasts for masses, and the fluid for cells. Some women routinely squeeze their nipples as part of their breast self-examination. This is unnecessary and may lead to an unimportant discharge.

Q. *I have been on the birth control pill for five years with no untoward symptoms. Recently I heard that some gynecologists think there may be a relationship between the Pill and breast cancer. Is that so?*

A. No, there is no definite evidence so far to incriminate the Pill in the development of breast cancer. The truth is that it will take some years before we may know definitely whether or not such pills could cause harm. In the meantime, most authorities agree that the possible danger from the Pill is considerably less than the medical risks of pregnancy. Any woman on the Pill should definitely have a complete breast examination at least once a year and be under the care of her gynecologist while taking it.

Q. *If I take hormones for the symptoms of menopause will they lead to breast cancer?*

A. There is some controversy about the use of female hormones in the menopause. Most authorities agree that these replacement hormones are harmless. Some feel strongly that hormones have a protective effect on the breast—that less breast cancer develops in women taking postmenopausal hormones. Some physicians feel equally strongly that this medication is dangerous and should not be used. Your best approach is to use hormones only when prescribed by your physician and to use them in the smallest dose necessary. Be sure to continue complete breast examinations.

Q. *What part does pregnancy play in breast cancer development? I have heard that women who have never been pregnant have a higher risk of developing breast cancer. Is this so?*

A. A woman who has had several children has a smaller chance of developing breast cancer than one who has never borne children. If a woman has a full-term child when she is under twenty years of age, her risk of developing breast cancer drops to one third of the usual risk. Pregnancy as such is not associated with breast cancer.

Since a woman who has had no children or one who
has her first child after the age of thirty has a slightly
increased risk of breast cancer, such women should definitely have the complete breast examination regularly.
Never, however, forget the monthly self-examination!

Q. *Is there any relationship between cancer and the shape,
size, and consistency of women's breasts?*

A. No. Cancer occurs in all types of breasts. It may
be more difficult to detect cancer earlier in very large
or very firm breasts. Until we find dependable high-
risk indicators, all women must be alert to the danger of breast cancer and learn the simple rules of
protection.

Q. *A year ago, while nursing my third child, I developed a
sore breast. It became red, hot, and painful, but gradually
subsided with medication. I still have some pain in this breast
and it is still firmer than my other breast. Is such a breast
more likely to develop a cancer?*

A. No. Inflammations, irritations, or infections in the
breast do not cause cancer, although residual lumps may
be present for a long time and will eventually disappear.
However, there is one unusual type of "inflammatory"
cancer which is not related to infection. This rare breast
cancer grows rapidly and may resemble a generalized
infection of the breast. Under any circumstances, definite breast lumps should be checked by a physician
promptly.

Q. *I've heard it said that it is good for the mother as well as
the child to nurse for six months or longer. While I was nursing*

my last child, my breasts dried up early. Is there any connection between this and the development of breast cancer?

A. No. We used to think that prolonged nursing protected against breast cancer. The latest data, however, indicate that it makes no difference whether a woman nurses at all or for long periods. It also makes no difference whether the breasts dry up naturally or with medication. To nurse or not to nurse is a question to be decided by you and your physician.

Q. *Is there any relationship between diet and breast cancer? Are overweight women more likely to develop breast cancer than those who are thin?*

A. We cannot prove that a relationship exists between diet and breast cancer. Some epidemiologists are convinced that increased risk of getting breast cancer is associated with a large intake of the kind of fats found in dairy food and beef. Some investigators think that an increase in saturated fats in the diet leads to increased production of female hormones and perhaps an increase in breast-cancer development. The increased numbers of breast cancer in those countries in which a substantial proportion of food intake is in saturated fats—as in northern Europe as compared with the Orient—is often cited as evidence. If a definite connection could be demonstrated, it might lead to another method of cancer control.

Q. *I have had cysts drained by my doctor in both breasts. It has been very disturbing to watch these large lumps reappear. Some of my friends have even had operations for this condition. Is there a connection between cysts and breast cancer?*

A. Many women have large breast lumps which develop rather quickly. They become extremely worried and then are reassured when the masses are found to have fluid which can be quickly and simply removed with a needle. Many women have cysts that require frequent examination. There is a difference of opinion among the experts as to whether large cysts induce a higher risk for breast-cancer development. An increased risk, if any, must be small or it would be obvious. Fortunately, large breast cysts tend to disappear after the menopause.

Large cysts usually do not constitute what is usually called "fibrocystic disease," a label that more often describes the lumpy texture of most normal breasts. This term refers to a vague, poorly defined entity which is probably not at all related to the development of breast cancer. It is usually used by physicians to describe a normal variation of breast consistency.

Q. *Is there any danger in having an annual examination of the breast in screening programs?*

A. No. Manipulation of the breast during regular clinical examination has potential benefit and no danger. Mammography uses X rays, but in expert hands and with modern methods, the dose needed is so minute that specialists agree that repeated examination is innocuous. Not having an examination, and possibly missing an early cancer, is certainly much more dangerous.

Q. *I am forty-two years old and have no breast symptoms. How often should I be examined?*

A. Every woman, including teenagers, should learn the details of breast self-examination and practice them regularly every month, preferably right after a period. After the menopause, the first of each month is an excellent time. Ask your physician to teach you how. A complete examination by a physician is advised once a year for all women over thirty-five. For the woman under thirty-five, mammography is not advised unless symptoms are present, particularly if she is at higher risk, or if she had a mother who developed breast cancer when she was menopausal.

Q. *My physician recommends that I report for examination every six months. Does this mean I am more likely to develop breast cancer?*

A. Many physicians recommend examinations more frequently than once a year. It certainly does not mean that a cancer is developing. It simply means that for medical reasons there may be a slightly increased risk and that they are taking extra precautions. This kind of special attention by a physician should be appreciated. Women needing more frequent examinations include those who (1) have already had a mastectomy; (2) have had breast operations; (3) have very large breasts; (4) have multiple, apparently benign large masses evident on clinical examination or on mammography; and (5) have a strongly positive family history, such as two or three close relatives with breast cancer.

Q. *Is a complete examination painful, tiring, or dangerous?*

A. Not at all. These procedures should not be painful. They are done quickly, and are completely without risk. Even mammography in expert hands uses so minute a dose of radiation that it can be repeated regularly for many years without risk. Usually, no injections or extra manipulations are used. The complete examination, including interview, clinical examination, and mammography, can be done in about twenty minutes.

Q. *I go to my gynecologist regularly once a year. He examines my breasts at that time. Is that enough of a breast examination?*

A. A complete examination as described in this book includes not only the clinical examination but also mammography. If your physician does not have the necessary equipment for some of these studies (as is usually the case), he may refer you to an appropriate source. Don't hesitate to ask about further studies. The increased reassurance of a complete examination using modern methods described in this book is well worth the extra time. It is most important for you to discuss breast self-examination with your gynecologist and have him go over the details with you.

Q. *Does breast cancer ever cure itself without treatment?*

A. It is extremely rare for breast cancer to be cured without treatment—if such remission occurs at all. Some advanced breast cancers are controlled by treatment as though a truce had been proclaimed. Occasionally, a woman may live for many years with breast cancer still present. For this reason no case of breast cancer should be considered hopeless.

Q. *My eighteen-year-old daughter found a small lump in her left breast three months ago. It has not changed since then. Could this become breast cancer? Should it be removed?*

A. Such lumps are common and cause concern, although only very rarely is such a mass serious. Each patient must be evaluated individually by the physician. Removal of these lumps is a simple procedure and often is the best answer. Occasionally, these masses, which are solid, not cysts filled with fluid, enlarge during pregnancy.

Q. *I have had a complete breast examination, including mammography and proper clinical examination, with completely negative report. Why do I have to continue such a study every year?*

A. It is generally agreed that breast cancer develops from a microscopic size when it cannot be detected by any of our sophisticated methods (even mammography) over a period of many years—up to ten years. This means that an examination may be completely negative but a cancer may still be developing. We must assume that this may be the case in every woman and that only a complete periodic study will be able to find it when it becomes detectable. Also, the risk increases with age so that screening for breast cancer is a lifelong necessity until we find the proper means to prevent the onset or development of the disease.

Q. *I have read in newspapers and magazines that some physicians tell women who have breast cancer that they have a right to enter into the decision regarding the type or extent of surgery to be performed. Is this correct?*

A. Yes; no operation can be done without the patient's consent. Since the most effective treatment for breast cancer is surgical, and since the breast is important in the psychology of women—and men—treatment should be discussed openly. Surgeons and their patients would prefer to have operations less extensive than mastectomy if they were proved to be effective. Unfortunately, there are no data that completely convince the general medical profession of the treatment needed for all individuals. The guiding principle in this situation fraught with emotional upheaval must be to consider the whole woman with cancer, rather than the cancer itself. Certainly, the surgeon about to perform a mastectomy understands the effects of that operation on the patient. It is the surgeon's responsibility to prevent emotional turmoil as much as possible, as well as to cure the disease. To do this, he or she should also discuss the problem in detail, with sympathy and understanding, with the husband as well as the patient. The surgeon must determine what is best for the emotional and the physical well-being of the patient. The woman, with her obvious lack of scientific knowledge about the type of treatment best for her particular problem, must rely on the advice of her personal physician and the surgeon. One thing is certain: The earlier the cancer is found, the better the outcome. When earlier breast-cancer detection becomes the rule, and not the exception as it is today, perhaps surgery less extensive than mastectomy may become the routine for more surgeons.

Q. *Do men get breast cancer?*

A. They do, but only one-hundredth as often as women. When it does occur, it is usually after the age of sixty. Because it is uncommon, men tend to neglect the findings until the disease is advanced. A man who finds a lump or any enlargement in his breast should observe the rules that apply to women.

GLOSSARY

acini The microscopic group of glands in the breast where milk is formed

areola The pigmented area around the nipple. Its size and prominence vary from individual to individual and change during one's lifetime. It contains several smaller raised areas which are tiny normal glands, called "Montgomery follicles."

axilla The armpit. It contains lymph glands or nodes, lymph channels, blood vessels, and fat. It has direct connections with the breast.

biopsy An operation of limited extent that removes a piece of breast for microscopic study and final diagnosis by a pathologist, a medical specialist trained in this type of examination

BSE Breast self-examination, or inspection and palpation of the breasts by the woman herself

chemotherapy Treatment using special chemicals which have the ability to destroy cancer cells

clinical examination Inspection and palpation of the breasts by a physician or by a trained paramedical person

death or mortality rate The number of deaths in relation to population numbers, usually given per 100,000 population

ducts The channels in the breast that lead from the acini to the nipple. The small passages are called ductules. These branch and end up in a group of six to fifteen large ducts that converge and open on the nipple. Their function is to convey the milk to the baby.

epidemiologist The specialist whose function is to gather data from many sources, often apparently unrelated, and use them to form explanations for the onset and development of diseases

estrogen One of the active female hormones that has a profound effect on the generative organs and breast. Its three main fractions are estradiol, estrone, and estriol.

fatty tissue Fat that acts as support and cushion for the delicate glandular tissue of the breast. After the menopause, most glandular tissue is replaced by fat.

fibrocystic disease A benign breast condition found in most women. It may vary in extent from minute microscopic cysts to large cysts filled with fluid. It accounts for the lumpy feeling that most breasts have. Aspiration of fluid or removal of a large cyst for microscopic tissue diagnosis may be in order. Fibrocystic disease itself probably has no connection with cancer.

fibrous tissue The firm supporting framework of the breast

glands A term used loosely to describe the functioning entity of many organs. The breast is referred to as a *mammary gland*. The lymph stations in the armpit are called *axillary lymph glands*, although they are actually lymph nodes. A *glandular system* refers to a group of glands having a similar function. The *endocrine glandular system* refers to that group of glands that produces hormones that have a widespread effect on the body, such as the ovaries, which are in the abdomen; the pituitary, which sits at the base of the brain; the thyroid, which rests on the trachea or windpipe; or the adrenals, which are located on top of the kidneys.

glandular tissue When referring to the breast, all of the acini where milk is produced

hormone therapy The use of hormones, or the substances produced by the endocrine glands, for treatment of breast diseases

immunotherapy The use of highly complex vaccines to stimulate the protective mechanism of the body, which is part of our defensive apparatus against disease or foreign substances

interview In a specialized sense, this term refers to the gathering of information from an individual about her family as well as her personal, educational, menstrual, childbearing, and breast history. Such data from large groups of women help to pinpoint those factors that are important in the initiation and development of disease and to identify the risk of developing breast cancer.

lumpectomy This is also called *partial mastectomy* or *tylectomy*. It is a surgical procedure in which only the breast cancer and a varying amount of breast tissue are removed as definitive treatment. The use of this procedure in the average woman has stirred a controversy among surgeons. It has an increasing number of adherents who advocate it under varying specified conditions, and a host of opponents who regard it as reprehensible.

lymphatic system An extensive network in the body which carries lymph. The lymphatic system has a series of many lymph nodes or way stations along its path that produce substances of immense benefit as part of the protective mechanism of the body against foreign material that produces disease. These lymph nodes act as a first line of defense in trapping cancer cells and destroying them. In breast cancer, the nodes most commonly involved are located in the armpit (the axillary nodes). Others are hidden under the breastbone (the internal mammary nodes) or above the collarbone (the supraclavicular nodes).

mammography A modern procedure which uses very small amounts of X rays to visualize the details of the breast structure. The examination is usually painless, quick, and easy. It takes but a few minutes and has become one of our most valuable studies because it gives us information about normal and abnormal changes in the breast tissues. The image produced is called a *mammogram*.

mastectomy Surgical removal of the breast. There are various techniques in which more or less tissue is removed at the same time. *Radical mastectomy*, which has been the procedure most commonly used, involves the removal of the chest muscles (pectoralis major and minor) together with the lymph nodes in the armpit. *Supraradical mastectomy* adds to the procedure the removal of nodes under the breastbone; this operation is done by its proponents for cancers close to the breastbone when involvement of these nodes is more likely. *Mod-*

ified radical mastectomy refers to a variation in which most of the chest muscles are left intact but the armpit nodes are removed. In this operation these latter glands usually cannot be removed as thoroughly as in the radical mastectomy. The procedure, however, results in substantially less deformity and makes it easier to construct a breast prosthesis for a more normal appearance. *Simple* or *total mastectomy* involves only removal of the breast, including its extension into the fold of the armpit, but does not include any substantial exploration of the armpit itself.

menopause The change of life, usually referring to the cessation of menstruation. It may have a gradual onset or be sudden. It is usually associated with physiological changes in the breast, with most of the breast structures eventually "involuting" or changing into fat.

metastasis A colony of cancer cells established away from its original source. The most common spread from breast cancer is to the local lymph nodes, the bones of the body, the liver, the lungs, or the brain. It is this tendency of cancer to metastasize that accounts for its deadly effect.

nodes Stations along the lymphatic channels of the body that defend neighboring organs from disease or contamination

pectoral muscles Muscular tissues attached to the chest wall and to the upper arms. These are divided into a larger group called pectoralis major, and a smaller group called pectoralis minor. Together they account for the fullness we see in the chest below the collarbones. There are some nodes in intimate contact with these muscles.

The muscles are removed totally or in part in the operation called radical mastectomy, primarily to make investigation of the armpit more thorough.

primary cancer Cancer arising initially in an organ— not as an extension or spread from a cancer at another site

radiation therapy The use of X rays in the treatment of disease, usually cancer. Various devices are used to produce these X rays. The apparatus used, such as an X-ray machine, a cobalt bomb, or various sophisticated and highly technical machines called linear accelerators, betatrons, etc., is responsible for the strength or penetrability of the X rays and varies with the special requirements of the cancer or the organ in which the cancer is situated. Basically, radiation therapy or X-ray treatment destroys rapidly growing cells, such as we find in cancer, more readily than it destroys normal cells. For this reason, such treatment is able to remove diseased cells without causing undue damage to surrounding normal cells.

secondary cancer Cancer developing in an organ as a result of the dissemination of a colony of cancer cells from a primary cancer elsewhere. Such a cancer is seeded by way of the bloodstream or the lymphatic channels.

specimen radiography The use of X rays to detect cancer in a biopsy specimen when it cannot be felt by the clinician. This procedure makes it possible to be sure that such a cancer has been removed and that the small area does indeed contain cancer cells. The area pinpointed by a specimen radiograph or X ray is then analyzed by the pathologist for a definite diagnosis. This procedure has proved to be invaluable in our attack on minimal or early breast cancer, which is often not palpable.

survival rate Refers to the percentage of women surviving a set period of time—such as five years—after a surgical procedure. It is often used by surgeons or radiotherapists in comparing one type of treatment with another. It has a built-in flaw, however: The survival rate depends on *when* in the course of the disease the cancer was first detected. Thus, a cancer found earlier through one method or another may indicate apparently longer survival, but actually the end result may be occurring at the same time as it would have if the cancer had been detected later. A better indicator is long-term survival rate of fifteen years or more. This would tend to equate with actual reduction of death rate or saving of lives.

tylectomy A more erudite synonym for *lumpectomy*

xeromammography A form of mammography in which the image produced by the X-ray machine is displayed on a Xerox selenium plate and subsequently transferred to a special paper, instead of using film.